# Rehabilitation after Severe Head Injury

*Dedication*

*This book is dedicated to the staff and patients of the Joint Services Medical Rehabilitation Unit, Royal Air Force, Chessington; and Rivermead Rehabilitation Centre, Oxford.*

# Rehabilitation after Severe Head Injury

EDITED BY

## C. D. Evans

MB BS MRCP(UK) DPhysMed
General Practitioner, Purley
Secretary of the International Rehabilitation Medicine
    Association, Basel, Switzerland
Formerly Consultant in Rheumatology and
    Rehabilitation, Oxford AHA(T)
Formerly Senior Medical Officer, Joint Services Medical
    Rehabilitation Unit, Royal Air Force, Chessington

CHURCHILL LIVINGSTONE
EDINBURGH LONDON MELBOURNE AND NEW YORK 1981

CHURCHILL LIVINGSTONE
Medical Division of Longman Group Limited

Distributed in the United States of America by Churchill
Livingstone Inc., 19 West 44th Street, New York, N.Y.
10036, and by associated companies, branches and
representatives throughout the world.

First published 1981

ISBN 0 443 01693 3

**British Library Cataloguing in Publication Data**
Rehabilitation after severe head injury.
  1. Head – Wounds and injuries
  I. Evans, C. D.
  617'.51    RD521

Printed in Hong Kong by
Wah Cheong Printing Press Ltd

# Preface

During the Second World War the Royal Air Force found that time spent in active rehabilitation of service personnel who had sustained injury paid considerable dividends. Such personnel returned to work quicker and fitter than those who had simply been sent home to recuperate on sick leave. During this period rehabilitation centres responded to the challenge of patients with orthopaedic injury such as multiple fractures, severe burns and other forms of trauma. After the war was over, a large number of the patients who passed through rehabilitation centres had sustained their injuries in road accidents rather than through active service, but it was still felt that the time spent in their rehabilitation was worthwhile. The fundamental principles laid down then have remained unchanged, but the extra experience gained and the new developments in therapy have been incorporated in contemporary rehabilitation centres. Many of the civilian centres set up over the last few years have derived much of their expertise and staff from those who have left the armed forces.

The pattern of injury, however, has also changed, as has the skill and care of management of patients in the acute stage. With the rapid development of accident and emergency services, and intensive treatment units, it is now possible for far more patients to survive the initial injury. Although this has led to an increased number of survivors from such injuries, it has also led to an increasing number of people who survive with severe handicap, and both service and civilian rehabilitation centres have had to respond to this challenge over the last 20 years. One particular area which has caused many problems throughout the world has been the management of those patients who have survived severe brain damage, but there is little that has been written about the long-term management and assessment even though it can be shown that the problem is increasing rather than decreasing at present.

This book is aimed to fill that gap and it reflects the practices at two rehabilitation centres, one being the Joint Services Medical Rehabilitation Unit at Royal Air Force Chessington, and the other

Rivermead Rehabilitation Centre in Oxford. The former unit can accommodate up to 200 patients of which the majority will be recovering from trauma but who have not sustained brain damage. However, between 20 and 30 patients at any one time may also be at this unit with the sequelae of brain damage. Rivermead Rehabilitation Centre is a smaller unit and can admit up to 46 patients, but out of this a large proportion have suffered brain damage, either from stroke or from head injury. Both units deal primarily with inpatients, though each has a small outpatient commitment in addition. Each unit admits over 50 brain-damaged patients a year and since the material in this book has been accumulated over about ten years, this represents observations on some 1000 patients. In addition, though not part of the material presented, there have been active research projects into assessment and management of brain damage, and these have had their effect on management as well.

All the contributors to the book have worked at one or the other of the two rehabilitation centres. Although each chapter is to some extent specialised, being written either by the therapist or doctor concerned with that subject, the contributors have had an awareness of the contributions to be made by other members of the team who shared the treatment of the patients and the writing of the book.

Since the book deals with the practice of these two units, it inevitably reflects the sort of cases that were admitted, so some aspects of rehabilitation after brain damage which might legitimately expect to find a place are not included since little experience was gained in their management. In particular, few cases of post-traumatic syndrome were encountered, so this has not formed a major part of the book. Nor through the stage of rehabilitation has epilepsy presented a major problem, though clearly when it comes to resettlement and discharge back into the community the presence or absence of epileptic attacks has an enormous bearing on employability and independence. But no attempt will be made in the book to cover this aspect of treatment. It aims instead to set down the practical management that was used and the approach made to some of the more severe and common problems encountered in rehabilitating patients after brain damage, and it is hoped that by adopting this approach each chapter will convey information for the profession that wrote it, and will also be comprehensible and valuable to those from other disciplines.

The editor would like to thank all the contributors for their work; the publishers for their forbearance; Mrs Ann White for typing (and retyping) the drafts, and the Director General of the Medical Services of the Royal Air Force for permission to publish.

*Surrey, 1981*                                                                 *C.D.E.*

# Contributors

**C. D. Evans** MB BS MRCP(UK) DPhysMed
(Chapters 1, 2 and 12)

**Elizabeth Rushworth** MB BS MRCP DCH    (Chapter 3)

**Meriel Davenport** LCST    (Chapter 4)

**Philippa Hall** LCST    (Chapter 4)

**Gillian Russell** BA (Squadron Leader, RAF)    (Chapter 5)

**Jane Stichbury** MCSP    (Chapter 6)

**Sue Whiting** MAOT    (Chapter 7)

**Ann Blackman** SRN    (Chapter 8)

**Gillian Walker** SRN    (Chapter 8)

**Nadina B. Lincoln** BSc MSc    (Chapter 9)

**Brian Key** MSRG DipTRG    (Chapter 10)

**Noel Gant** MSRG DipTRG    (Chapter 10)

**Elizabeth Trumble** BSc CQSW    (Chapter 11)

The contributors all worked either at the Joint Services Medical Rehabilitation Unit, Royal Air Force, Chessington or at Rivermead Rehabilitation Centre, Oxford during the course of the work which is described in this book.

# Contents

# 1

# The epidemiology of head injury, and the assessment of its severity and consequences

## INTRODUCTION

One of the most significant growth points in medicine over the last 20 years has been the quality of care given to victims of severe accidents or other episodes in which there has been cerebral damage. The advance has taken place not only in the accident and emergency services but in the initial care at the roadside, in transportation and in intensive treatment units within hospitals, and consequently there has been an increase in the number of survivors of head injury.

London (1967) estimated that there were 700 to 800 'lame brains' who survived each year in England and Wales, and no figures published subsequently suggest that this was an overestimate. Field (1976) produced a comprehensive review of the epidemiology of head injury in addition to reviewing contemporary research. He drew his figures from the *Hospital In-Patient Enquiry* (HIPE), which is published by the Department of Health and Social Security. The HIPE is the analysis of a 1-in-10 sample of all patients who are discharged from or die in hospital in England and Wales each year, although because of the time taken for analysis the figures are inevitably some two or three years in arrears. From Table 1.1 it will be seen that in 1975 about 150 000 patients were discharged from hospitals with the diagnosis of intracranial injury or concussion. The staggering statistics are due to the large number of people admitted with minor head injury, perhaps sustained in a fight or a fall or minor

**Table 1.1** Estimated total discharges and deaths in 1975 with mean duration of stay (MDS), nature of injury and place of occurrence
AN 143
Intracranial injury (not fracture)

| RTA | | Home | | Other, unspecified | | Total | |
|---|---|---|---|---|---|---|---|
| Est. No. | MDS | Est. No. | MDS | Est. No. | MDS | Est. No. | MDS |
| 33 000 | 4.5 | 19 490 | 4.1 | 69 420 | 3.1 | 121 910 | 3.6 |
| *Concussion* | | | | | | | |
| 8 420 | 3.7 | 3 230 | 4.4 | 14 870 | 2.8 | 26 250 | 3.3 |
| | | | | | | Total 148 | 430 |

1

road traffic accident. The overwhelming majority of these patients make an uninterrupted and uneventful recovery, though a significant minority who appear to have suffered little damage do in the long term complain of sequelae, so forming another group which is the subject of considerable study. Some cases in this group become labelled as the 'post-traumatic syndrome', or 'post-concussional syndrome', and whether the cause of the condition is organic or functional is still being debated. The truth probably is that within the group there are some people who have sustained significant organic lesions that we are not yet able to detect and that in others poor motivation or impending litigation turns what should have been a trivial injury into a major handicap. Sometimes it is hard not to suspect the active participation by the patient, his relatives, legal advisers, or at least that the situation is condoned by these groups and indeed the caring staff. Sometimes this is done deliberately and other times probably unconsciously. Table 1.1 also shows that the mean duration of stay for these patients was over three days, so this group represents a considerable drain on hospital resources. Furthermore, this table excludes all those patients who sustained fracture, a group which, though not numerically large, would add to the total still further. The importance of the minor lesion is therefore not to be underestimated but is not within the scope of the book. Work being undertaken at Oxford (Newcombe et al 1979) is beginning to shed light on the sort of damage that is being sustained and its practical sequelae. Cohadon (1974) feels that an aggressive policy of rehabilitation for such patients does pay dividends though the problems attendant upon detailed research and the problems of carrying out adequate control trials make hard evidence difficult to come by.

Figure 1.1 gives an analysis of the discharge rates for 1974 and it can be seen that there are two peaks of incidence of head injury, one peak relates to patients between the ages of 15 and 19 years and the other to the elderly, i.e. those who are over 75 years. It also shows that in the younger age group men are much more at risk than women, and that overall men are twice as likely to sustain head injury than women, though the difference becomes less marked towards the later part of life. The HIPE study also analyses the discharges and deaths of children under 15 years (Fig. 1.2) and the figures show that for both sexes the vulnerable age is between 5 and 9 years. As this is only a 1-in-10 sample, the figures need to be treated with caution, but it does in general confirm what common sense would suggest, i.e. that the overwhelming majority of accidents are to young men, and that road traffic accidents and home accidents are the two most important causes of these injuries. In addition to the 800 or so 'lame brains', it is

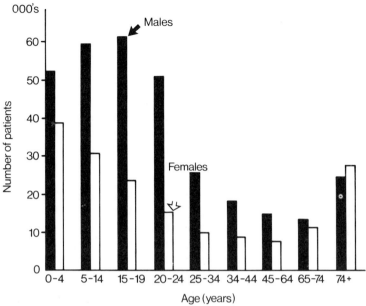

**Fig. 1.1**    Discharge rates per 10 000 population: sex, age group and diagnostic groups
for 1974.

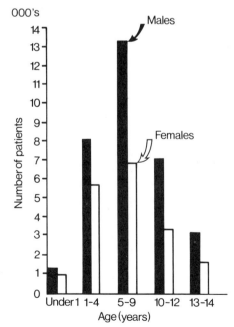

**Fig. 1.2**    Estimated total discharges and deaths of children under 15 years of age: sex,
age and selected diagnostic groups.

estimated that there are several thousand more patients each year who are rendered incapable of following their original occupations. Many of these people return to the community where they can totally disrupt a family. Others may end in inappropriate placements within hospitals, either in the psychogeriatric unit as being one of the few places who will care for them, and still others will end up equally misplaced in a wide variety of institutions ranging from voluntary organisations such as the Cheshire Foundation, in hostel accommodation or tucked away in an obscure corner in the general hospital to which they were first admitted after the accident. There can be very few acute hospitals within the United Kingdom that do not harbour one or two such patients.

If long-term residential care is the outcome, the cost (1979) for each patient could ultimately be of the order of £400 000 since the majority of survivors are young and they might live another 30 or 40 years and it is very difficult to find accommodation which provides full care for the dependent patient which costs less than £100 to £125 per week. For those patients who are misplaced in general hospitals the cost is far higher, but for all the increased cost it does not mean that such patients are getting appropriate or indeed any treatment relevant to their condition.

The challenge facing rehabilitation centres that deal with the brain-damaged survivor is to lighten the load of dependency as much as possible. Obviously the ideal to be striven for is normality, but in practical terms for many patients this is not going to be achieved. In this case the staff who care for such patients need to know the length of time when active rehabilitation should be pursued, what form it should take, how often it should be given and when its usefulness cannot be considered any more to be cost-effective. Similar questions can be asked of the management of survivors from stroke. Unfortunately research methods involving control trials are difficult to set up, time-consuming and expensive to run, and for this reason the amount of information that can be given with confidence is very small, and even now the amount of hard evidence that has emerged to guide doctors, therapists and relatives in caring for their handicapped patient is still limited.

Head injury, therefore, is extremely common and although most cases are relatively mild, within the United Kingdom each year there are several thousand people who are going to be expensive to the community both in their consumption of time and money, and it was the realisation of this that was the stimulus to the research referred to later in the book.

ASSESSMENT

It became apparent during the early 1970s that the rehabilitation units of the services were having to deal with the brain-damaged survivor in numbers that they had not met before. Earlier reports by Lewis (1966) and Knight (1973) had discussed the management of patients with brain damage, and awareness of the sharp increase in the numbers being admitted initiated a long-term research project into how best to handle and retrain the survivors for independence. There being very little practical information available to guide doctors and therapists in the best technique available, it was decided to try to improve the assessment of the severity of the original head injury and the physical, psychological and mental sequelae that the survivors had sustained. It was also deemed important that those who spent most of their time dealing with the day to day problems of such patients should be asked to contribute their own assessment so that everyone would bring an individual approach to the task. In devising the basic assessment, some arbitrary decision had to be taken about the topics which would be assessed and treated by which department. Some areas were chosen deliberately, others by design and some of the omissions of the original scheme were not from choice but from lack of availability of staff to undertake the tests. The assessment that was done by the departments was designed to concentrate on identifying the problems that had been left after the head injury had taken place and the patient had been admitted to the rehabilitation centre, but in addition to this some consideration had to be given to the measurement and assessment of the original damage sustained by the brain.

The only available information on the assessment of the severity of the original injury was based on the study by Ritchie Russell and Smith (1961), who used the duration of post-traumatic amnesia as the criterion for assessing the severity of the original injury (see Table 1.2). It rapidly became apparent that for the group of patients being admitted that this measure was not going to be relevant, partly because many of the patients were still in post-traumatic amnesia (PTA) when they arrived and partly because PTA can only ever be a retrospective measurement. Since our intention was to predict the outcome of brain

Table 1.2 Grading of the severity of a head injury

| 0 | PTA | Nil |
|---|---|---|
| 1 | PTA less than 1 hour | Mild |
| 2 | PTA more than 1 hour, less than 1 day | Moderate |
| 3 | PTA more than 1 day, less than 1 week | Severe |
| 4 | PTA more than 1 week | Very severe |

**Table 1.3**  Duration of post-traumatic amnesia

|  | Number of patients |
|---|---|
| Less than 1 hour | 0 |
| More than 1 hour but less than 24 hours | 4 |
| More than 1 day but less than 1 week | 13 |
| More than 1 week but less than 2 weeks | 9 |
| More than 2 weeks but less than 3 weeks | 12 |
| More than 3 weeks but less than 4 weeks | 7 |
| More than 4 weeks but less than 5 weeks | 8 |
| More than 5 weeks but less than 6 weeks | 0 |
| More than 6 weeks but less than 7 weeks | 4 |
| More than 7 weeks but less than 8 weeks | 3 |
| More than 8 weeks but less than 12 weeks | 5 |
| More than 12 weeks but less than 16 weeks | 3 |
| More than 16 weeks but less than 20 weeks | 5 |
| More than 20 weeks but less than 24 weeks | 0 |
| 24 weeks + | 19 |
| N K | 7 |
| N R | 4 |
|  | Total   103 |

damage it was clear that this definition would be inadequate for our purposes. Table 1.3 shows the duration of PTA recorded for the 103 patients who were studied at Chessington.

It was therefore decided to add the duration of unconsciousness as a measure of severity of the initial injury (Table 1.4). The definition was derived from the work of Plum and Posner (1972) and corresponded closely to the definitions being used in Glasgow in a similar study in patients with severe brain damage. This latter work has demonstrated that the duration and depth of coma are good predictors not only of survival but to broad categories of outcome. This sets a standard for

**Table 1.4**  Duration of unconsciousness

|  | Number of patients |
|---|---|
| Less than 1 hour | 4 |
| More than 1 hour but less than 24 hours | 12 |
| More than 1 day but less than 3 days | 8 |
| More than 3 days but less than 1 week | 20 |
| More than 1 week but less than 2 weeks | 12 |
| More than 2 weeks but less than 3 weeks | 11 |
| More than 3 weeks but less than 4 weeks | 3 |
| More than 4 weeks but less than 8 weeks | 9 |
| More than 8 weeks but less than 12 weeks | 10 |
| 12 weeks + | 3 |
| N K | 9 |
| N R | 2 |
|  | Total   103 |

those involved in rehabilitation to see whether by specialised techniques of retraining, the quality of life of the survivors can be improved.

## Definitions
*Post-traumatic amnesia.* This was defined as 'the duration of the loss of memory from the time of the original injury to the time when continual day to day memory has been re-established'. *Unconsciousness.* This is from the time of injury to the time when a patient can make a meaningful response which is better than 'Yes' or 'No' but which takes into account the limits of speech which might be imposed by mechanical factors such as tracheostomy or a wired jaw.

Inquiry was also made regarding retrograde amnesia but in the group of patients under study it seemed to contribute little and although recorded was subsequently abandoned as a predictor.

The duration of unconsciousness and post-traumatic amnesia was recorded as accurately as possible from notes, patients, relatives and any other available source. Note was taken of whether alcohol had been involved at the time of the injury. If the cause of the injury had been a road traffic accident, the category of the patient was also recorded, i.e. unprotected road user, driver, or passenger (Table 1.5). A full record was made of any associated injury and operations, particularly if such might have influenced the apparent duration of unconsciousness. This information was picked up usually in the initial discussions with the medical officer and the patient and relatives, supplemented by information from the notes.

**Table 1.5** Analysis of type of road user

|                      | Good outcome | Moderate outcome | Poor outcome | Total |
|----------------------|:---:|:---:|:---:|:---:|
| Vehicle driver       | 13 | 4 | 6 | 23 |
| Vehicle passenger    | 9  | 4 | 6 | 19 |
| Motorcycle driver    | 2  | 9 | 1 | 12 |
| Motorcycle passenger | 1  | — | — | 1  |
| Unprotected road user| 8  | 3 | 9 | 20 |
| N K                  | 1  | 1 | 3 | 5  |
| Total                | 34 | 21 | 25 | 80 |

## Assessment of the consequences of injury
Assessment is only useful if it is being done with a specific purpose in mind. Throughout the country an enormous amount of assessments are done formally; through clinical or other examination, or informally through ordinary patient-staff contact. Many of these produce

unrecordable information and many others produce no useful information since no relevant question was asked. For example, it is reasonable to ask an occupational therapist to assess a patient to see if he is capable of self-care at home; but the question is irrelevant if the social conditions there would prevent his return anyway.

It was decided that the therapeutic departments should design their own assessments and, as referred to already, although these allowed of some overlap, where this has occurred it has been usually deliberate. It may also seem from reading the individual chapters that these assessments take a great deal of time to do and that a lot of trouble was taken both in their making and recording. This point will be taken up in the individual chapters concerned, and it will be shown that the tests are not as time-consuming as they initially appear to be, since they could be done while treatment was being carried out.

In designing assessments the four factors of repeatability, relevance, recordability and retrievability were borne in mind, otherwise it is extremely easy to end up with a laboriously compiled set of notes which will convey no useful information. Therefore a system of scoring was devised for each department, which though not without its faults has at least permitted some comparison and standardisation to be undertaken. The education department in particular had one special advantage, shared to a lesser extent by the other department, in that a great deal was known about the educational and physical abilities of the Service patient from before the accident. This made research into the handicap caused by the accident a great deal more realistic.

**Repeatability**
It must not matter which therapist in the department has undertaken a particular assessment but in order to do so they have to be trained and interobserver studies undertaken in order to see the level of error that may be expected between observers. Here the use of closed-circuit television allows comparisons to be made without inconvenience to the patient. Recent studies undertaken at Rivermead Rehabilitation Centre by Lincoln & Leadbitter (1979) and Whiting & Lincoln (1980) show their careful assessment of functional ability and also the lengths to which these therapists went in order to identify and then reduce observer error. This programme involved the use of videotape both for training observers and storing information, as well as Guttman scales (see Chapter 9).

**Relevance**
There are two widely disparate reasons for initiating formal assessments, one being concerned with research and the other

concerned with the practical aspect of the patient's care. In the former case, particularly, observations need to be precise since change has to be identified clearly. In doing so it has to be also accepted that much information may be sought which will subsequently prove to be redundant; but provided this type of assessment is not confused with the second group then problems need not arise. It is difficult, however, to persuade therapists who are primarily concerned with the service commitment for the handicapped patient to do prolonged investigations which seem futile to the therapist, however important it may be to the researcher. (It was largely for this reason that the therapists themselves were invited to design their own assessments.)

In the event the two aims need not be incompatible and a well-designed research assessment may also help therapists to produce better practical assessments than the less formal ones.

## Recordability

Subjective narrative reports may mislead and are certainly time-consuming though not entirely dispensable. It is possible to devise or use existing systems of scored assessments where answers to the question of ability are scored on a level of 0 to 5. Other questionnaires can be done on a straight yes/no basis and both techniques were used both in Oxford and in Chessington. Not surprisingly, other workers have confirmed that the more choices that are left open for decisions the bigger the scatter between observers, and a 0 to 5 scale seems at present to be the one most universally used. Many of the questionnaires produced for assessment of the ability for activities of daily living were reviewed by Donaldson (1974). She came to the conclusion also that it was confusing to offer more than a five-point scale for any given activity. However, the problem can be solved by phrasing the questions in a different way and in Figure 1.3 the alternative systems are shown. In the first one the choice has to be made of one out of five, but in the second a series of true/false questions are asked and again this has validity since it can show change, but does not ask the therapist to be forced into an apparently impossible decision.

## Retrievability

Figure 1.4 shows a summary chart of information on one patient. It will be clear that a large amount of information is easy to obtain and it is also possible to get workable material from it. With more modern methods of information processing such data are storable on a computer. In the study under discussion this facility was not available but the material was also suitable for graphic display. Figure 1.5 shows

A

JOINT POSITION SENSE

Information can be recorded on a graded scale,

Score 0 – 5

|  | Right | Left |
|---|---|---|
| Metatarso-phalangeal joints |  |  |

Scale of Grading

0 = Unaware of movement

1 = Aware at extremes only

2 = Aware of gross movement (>60°)

3 = Aware of coarse movement (>30°)

4 = Aware of fine movement ( >10°)

5 = Normal                              or . . . . . . . . . .

B

JOINT POSITION SENSE

As a series of True/False choices.
The metatarso-phalangeal joint of the right foot has:

|  | True | False |
|---|---|---|
| No awareness of movement |  |  |
| Awareness at extremes only |  |  |
| Aware of gross movement (>60°) |  |  |
| Aware of coarse movement (>30°) |  |  |
| Aware of fine movement ( >10°) |  |  |
| Normal |  |  |

**Fig. 1.3** Alternative methods of recording information.

further change recorded for the same patient over the next five years.

The development of more formal hierarchical systems of recovery is discussed in the chapters on clinical psychology and future developments. It is worth emphasising here the point that if recovery is known to take place in a given sequence, then planning treatment programmes becomes a much more realistic exercise. This is because the aim of therapists is to produce a task for the patient which is neither beneath his dignity nor beyond his competence. Such planning can follow these assessments.

Up to this point this chapter has been concerned with an attempt to identify the scale of the problem and to outline the reasons behind the development of both general and specific assessments, both of the severity of the original head injury and of its sequelae. It is also important to have a clear idea of what rehabilitation is attempting to do, and in order to do this some definition of rehabilitation needs to be given.

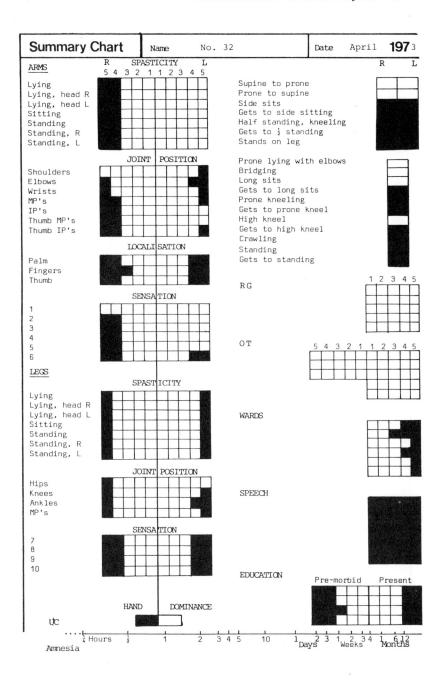

**Fig. 1.4**  Summary chart of patient on admission.

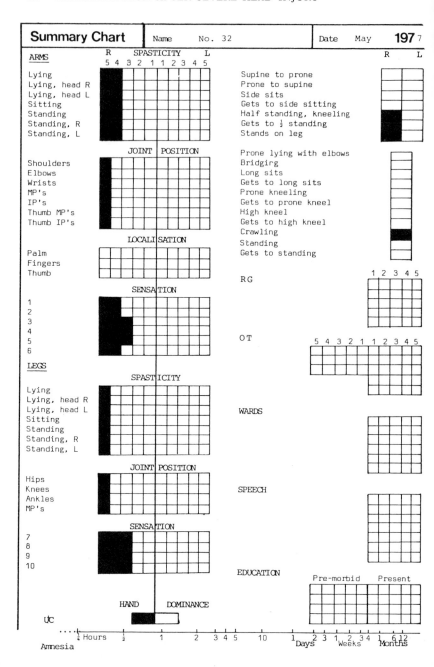

**Fig. 1.5**   Summary chart of same patient after five years.

*Rehabilitation.* This can be regarded as the reintegration of the patient with his original environment. This is a brief definition and was given anonymously by a medical student but it draws attention to the three aspects which are important, namely the patient himself, the need for reintegration and the importance of studying the environment from which the patient originally came. It is also possible to regard rehabilitation from three different points of view, the first being that of manipulating the physical or mental condition of the patient by therapeutic endeavour. The second is to adapt the environment to which the patient will return and the third is to alter the attitudes both of the patient and those who will have to care for him upon his return into the community or in his absorption into another environment. It is possible to find units which concentrate on one perhaps to the exclusion of the other two aspects, but in considering the rehabilitation of patients after brain damage it is of crucial importance to examine all three possible routes of achieving final reintegration.

REFERENCES

Cohadon F 1974 From papers read at the International Conference on Head Injury held in Oslo in 1974
Donaldson S W 1973 A unified ADL form. Archives of Physical Medicine and Rehabilitation 54: 175-179
Field J H 1975 A study of the epidemiology of head injury in England and Wales, with particular reference to rehabilitation. (A report to the DHSS)
Knight P N 1972 Rehabilitation of head injury. Nursing Mirror March: 14-18
Lewis N R 1966 Rehabilitation after head injury. Proceedings of the Royal Society of Medicine 59: 623-625
Lincoln N B, Leadbitter D 1979 Assessment of motor function in stroke patients. Physiotherapy 65: 48-51
London P S 1967 Some observations in the course of events after severe injuries of the head. (Hunterian Lecture.) Annals of the Royal College of Surgeons of England 41: 460
Newcombe F, Artiola I, Fortuna L 1979 Problems and perspectives in the evaluation of psychological deficits after cerebral lesions. International Rehabilitation Medicine 1: 182-192
Plum F, Posner B 1972 Diagnosis of stupor and coma, 2nd edn. Davis, Philadelphia
Russell W R, Smith R 1961 PTA in closed head injury. Archives of Neurology 5: 4
Whiting S E, Lincoln N B 1980 Assessment of activities of daily living in stroke patients. British Journal of Occupational Therapy Feb: 44-46

# 2

# The organisation of a rehabilitation centre

In most rehabilitation centres representatives of most of the following professions will be found. Since their interaction is so crucial, a short paragraph on each of the disciplines will be given. Lists of members of a team are always open to the danger that somebody crucial will be omitted, so that although this is intended to be a list of all the relevant likely disciplines, some group may have been left off, in which case profound apologies are offered. It will be noted by the discerning reader that the list is in alphabetical order and this was deliberate so as not to imply a hierarchy, though of course the hierarchy within a rehabilitation team and unit is one which will evolve and under no circumstances must be taken for granted.

## CLINICAL PSYCHOLOGISTS

Usually these have an academic background and a university degree. According to Chambers dictionary, psychology is the study of mind and behaviour, so the psychologist's role in the rehabilitation of patients with brain damage is crucial. In practical terms the clinical psychologist is expected to be able to make formal definitions and assessments of such qualities as memory, mood, intellect, comprehension and expression. All are of great moment both to the attendants and relatives of those who have suffered brain damage. In most departments there are insufficient number of clinical psychologists to do all the work that could be set before them, so that frequently they are left with the unhappy task of being asked to do assessments but are unable to give any form of therapeutic help as a consequence of their assessments. It is a rare unit where the establishment for clinical psychologists is large enough for them to make a significant contribution to treatment. When such contributions are possible, then the setting of realistic goals, behaviour modification, introducing suitable incentives for patients (and sometimes for their relatives and staff), can be undertaken. In many units there is no establishment for a clinical psychologist at all, and

14

then their role is partly taken over by speech therapists and occupational therapists.

## DISABLEMENT RESETTLEMENT OFFICERS (DROs)

These officials are not members of the National Health Service but responsible to the Department of Employment. The DROs provide invaluable support in the rehabilitation of many categories of handicapped patients, including those with brain damage. If there is likely to be a problem in re-employment, then the earlier that the help of the DRO can be invoked the better. Should it later become apparent that the patient may be able to get back his original job, suitable pre-training courses may still have to be arranged. If a change of job appears inevitable, then the Employment Medical Advisory Service can also be contacted through the DRO, and a wide range of assessment and training and help with employment can be given. Money can be provided for courses which are not available in Government Training Centres (Skill Centres). Recruitment of the DRO early on will help to minimise, even eliminate, the delay between the time the patient leaves hospital or rehabilitation centre and the time he starts work. A long period of delay before starting work is very destructive to morale for the vast majority of those patients for whom work has previously been part of their ethic. However, with the present high levels of unemployment and probability of routine jobs being lost in the future, it may be that resettlement of the handicapped into work will become much more difficult and resettlement into constructive retirement will become the norm.

## DOCTORS

The role of the doctor during the phase of rehabilitation has always been to some extent equivocal, and is undergoing change at present. There seems to be no alternative but that he is legally responsible for the general care and direction of rehabilitation effort, though which doctor has this task is not always clear. For example, during the acute stage, while the patient is in hospital, then the overall management is the responsibility of the neurosurgeon, orthopaedic surgeon or general surgeon in whose department the patient is, but once the patient has left hospital and gone home, or is attending a rehabilitation centre, then the responsibility becomes divided. Furthermore, because of the original doctor's main role, which will involve him in much routine medical work, there is little time to take a direct interest in the rehabilitation after the acute stage. This responsibility is then delegated, formally or informally, either to junior medical staff, who quite frequently have little experience or interest in the field, or it may go to therapists or to the general practitioner. The first option is undesirable, but if the second channel is to be adopted then it needs to be done formally so that in the event of medical advice being required, the place to get it is clear. Until the last few years it has been tacitly assumed that the doctor heads the rehabilitation team. However with the rising status of senior therapeutic staff, this assumption is no longer valid and there will be situations in which the doctor is regarded either as a screen to ensure that there is no medical condition which needs treatment or as a source of advice. The admission, discharge and day-to-day handling of the patient then ceases to be his responsibility and is assumed, de facto, by another member of the team.

## NURSES

The role of the nurse in rehabilitation is also changing rapidly. There was a time when the ward sister and nursing staff assumed the responsibility for all the day-to-day management of the patient. A few years ago the ward sister would organise voluntary and other forms of help to do what other therapists are now asked to do. Social enquiry, talking to relatives and the preparation for the patient's discharge, would also have been the nurse's responsibility. With proliferation of other rehabilitation staff, this is now not always so. Where a clear allocation of responsibility has been agreed, problems are trivial, but where it is unresolved, duplication of effort and conflicting advice can result. Conflict may occur at many levels, but the link of greatest importance is the one between the therapists and the nursing staff. The therapeutic staff may decide that a given form of physical treatment should be adopted (and there are many systems available, all with their special advantages claimed), e.g. there is universal agreement in the departments that one system of lifting is to be used, while a totally different form of treatment is used in the wards. This will cause uncertainty from the patient's and relatives' point of view: it is feasible, though, and essential, for the therapists to spend time ensuring that members of the nursing staff are aware of the current system. They can help to explain why particular techniques of lifting, sitting, posturing and feeding should be adopted. (In a really dedicated unit, the therapists will come in late at night in order that the night staff shall then share this information as well.) Then, when the treatment programme becomes consistent, better results seem to be achieved, though as with many other problems in rehabilitation, establishing this to be statistically significant is difficult.

Frequently, in tasks such as dressing and feeding, it is quicker to do the work for the patient rather than wait while he attempts to do it himself. This is an unfortunate truth, and it seems that if the nurses are to play their full part in the rehabilitation effort their establishment must be such as to allow more time with patients; then work in departments is able to be carried on through the evenings and weekends.

## OCCUPATIONAL THERAPISTS

The occupational therapists train over a three-year period, and have a working knowledge of anatomy, physiology and medical conditions and some knowledge of craft work. Recently they seem to have specialised in assessment of activities of daily living (ADL), provision of aids, and in some instances, into the assessment of basic psychological problems. The Association of Occupational Therapists is running courses to train OTs to administer some of the basic psychological tests which hitherto have been administered only by clinical psychologists. This is a constructive development since it is unrealistic to expect that all hospitals can establish clinical psychologists in the foreseeable future. Because of the number of hospital departments in which occupational therapy is available, the therapists play a significant part in the rehabilitation of patients with brain damage, and are often called in to give the final assessment before attempting to discharge the patient home into the community. Some progressive departments are also assessing perceptual problems and making active strides to overcome such deficits. Where this facility is available then it is usually invoked as early as possible in the rehabilitation of the patient. In this book, the role of the occupational therapist in perceptual assessment and retraining will be particularly stressed.

## PHYSIOTHERAPISTS

This profession has a three year course, at the end of which the physiotherapist is expected to have a working knowledge of general anatomy and physiology, with a detailed coverage of the musculoskeletal and nervous systems. Over the last few years some members of this profession have spent a great deal of time in the development of assessments of physical ability. Physiotherapy departments both in the United Kingdom and overseas have been responsible for many different systems of physical rehabilitation — Bobath methods being just one such system. In some of the systems under use, the neurophysiological basis has always seemed somewhat sketchy, but as to which system is best it seems that the conviction of the therapist that what he or she is doing is correct is probably of more significance than the actual technique itself. Where a department decides on a specific technique then, as has already been stressed, all other disciplines must be made aware of this decision and respect it. Frequently the introduction of a system necessitates close collaboration between the therapy departments, and this in itself leads to what, in contemporary jargon, is called the 'integrated team approach'.

## RELATIVES

Some of the reasons why relatives should be included as part of the therapy team are sufficiently obvious to require mention but no elaboration. For somebody with severe brain damage, the people most likely to be left with the major responsibility and problem are the relatives, and a tremendous amount of cooperation and help must be given if they are to have any prospect of success in this very difficult task. The chance of success depends not only on the severity of the injury but on which relative it is who subsequently has to look after the victim. The prospects of satisfactory return home appear greatest when the injured themselves are young and where the mother is still able to care. If only the father is available, then the chance of a successful return home is smaller. If the patients themselves are older, and the relatives are elderly, then returning a patient home is often an unstable solution, because with increasing frailty either the mother or father, or both parents, are unable to cope and then another placement has to be sought. It is also difficult to resettle an elderly patient with brain damage on to their children for a long time, particularly if there is a young family as well. Even moderate social handicap turns this into an unacceptable position. It may sometimes be possible with planned support, holiday relief and other forms of social and medical aid, to ease the load on the caring relatives. If so, these aids should be used as early as possible to help the whole family to achieve stability.

Relatives can be of major value much earlier. The presence of relatives beside the bed helps the newly injured to re-establish contact with reality and to learn what has happened. Proof of this statement in statistical terms is impossible, but many brain-damaged survivors have been able to recall precisely information that was being given them during the time when they appeared to be unconscious and uncommunicative. They recall this attention with deep gratitude and affection. On a completely commonsense basis, it appears a reasonable course of action, and in practical terms it is usually encouraged by all acute units. One group of relatives introduced a visitors' book after the first two days on the ward where each relative or friend who came noted the date and the subject of any conversation that they may have had with the patient, and any observations that they were able to make with special reference to what was known about the patient from before the accident. Since this information is so rarely available, this book, charting the recovery of the patient from deep coma, provided a tremendous insight for the nursing and medical staff on the ward concerned. It seems a simple and useful way of gathering information and involving the relatives from a very early stage in the programme of rehabilitation. It also permitted much more communication between the nursing staff and the relatives than normally can be guaranteed.

## REMEDIAL GYMNAST

To the outside observer this discipline has a great deal in common with physiotherapy. Often the similarities in task are more apparent than the differences. There are historical reasons why the two professions should have grown up separately, and other reasons why they are unable to merge. Numerically there are far fewer remedial gymnasts than physiotherapists and in general terms their work is designed more to the administration of physical exercise than to the application of electrically or other physically based treatments. However, with the move away from such treatments by the physiotherapists and the adoption by remedial gymnasts of the skills to give basic heat and ice therapy, the differences have become even fewer. In practice their recruitment and involvement in the team of a rehabilitation unit depends more on local history and staff availability than anything else, and the role in which they are used is similarly unpredictable. In the later stages of rehabilitation they may get themselves more involved with class work; even this generalisation is disputable, but in the context of the services, then their role is more specific, and merits a separate chapter.

## REHABILITATION ENGINEERS

Few units will have the services of such a professional, it being almost inevitable that at the present time they are confined to research units and university departments. However, if these specific services are not available and some item of equipment has to be individually made, there are alternative sources available, and one such in the United Kingdom is REMAP, whose address is given in the Appendix.

## SOCIAL WORKER

Administratively, social workers are no longer part of the health care team since they are employed by the local authority, and subsequently seconded to work in hospitals or rehabilitation centres. Being a relatively new discipline the contribution that they have to make is capable still of being misunderstood. For example, nursing staff may feel that making contact with relatives and counselling was originally part of their role and are reluctant to transfer that responsibility, although in the vast majority of cases they have not the time to do it justice. Again, the social worker frequently has the time to listen to apparently minor, non-medical problems of the patients and relatives and can form a better relationship than doctors or other staff involved. The shortage of time is usually quoted as the reason why involvement falls off, but it is imperative that somebody takes this responsibility, and it usually devolves upon the social worker. Provided case conferences are taken seriously and communication is good, no insoluble problem arises; but this is another area where contacts can fail, and once more the sufferer is the patient (or, if they are the responsibility of the social work department, the client!). To some extent the impatience which is occasionally felt is generated by the somewhat Panglossian attitude that some social workers may have. Other professionals can see more clearly where their responsibility ends, but the social worker knows that he or she will be the person who, next to the relatives, will have the biggest responsibility for the longest period of time, once the patient has left hospital. They also frequently find themselves the unenviable buffer between relatives and medical staff. This can be very trying when the hospital or rehabilitation centre is trying to discharge a patient and the social worker can see only too clearly the problems that are involved in this manoeuvre. Return to the community based on a consistent team approach, liaison with the available community services, and a gradual transition, possibly by allowing the patient home at weekends only, or during the week, can encourage the relatives to take over in many cases. Resettlement often has to be supervised by the social work department, which will also be responsible for ensuring that any statutory help is provided and that the necessary adaptations to the home and work are undertaken and paid for.

## SPEECH THERAPISTS

This profession has evolved greatly over the last few years, but for wide areas of the United Kingdom the amount of staff available is only token. Where this situation obtains, the most profitable role for the therapist is to assess at what level communication with the patient exists and how the relatives and nursing staff may in fact capitalise upon what comprehension and expression there is. In the absence of both the speech therapist and a clinical psychologist, the responsibility for this particular function may devolve upon the occupational therapist. Rest somewhere it must, for establishment of any method of communication as early as possible with the brain-damaged survivor seems to be of crucial importance. As in cases of stroke, it would appear that perception of hearing and seeing precede recovery in expression by a considerable time. In theory, this information is widely known: in practice it is frequently forgotten, and the patient can easily become the equivalent of a pillow in the bed to be talked over, and around, but never to. Patients who recover after a long time comment on this, often in terms of the strongest resentment. In later stages of recovery, when speech may be relatively normal but articulation slow and confusing, it is again of the utmost importance that the response of the therapeutic staff and the relatives should be to treat the patient as having a normal perception and comprehension, even if the evidence appears to point to the contrary. There is little to be lost by such a strategy and everything to be gained.

## TECHNICAL INSTRUCTORS

Technical instructors may supervise retraining, either for an original job or a suitable alternative. It is unlikely that these staff will be present in many hospitals, but they are represented in some rehabilitation centres. There needs to be close liaison between them and the occupational therapy department. In a few hospitals the instructors are actually part of such a department.

Although assessments carried out by technical instructors in hospital and rehabilitation centres have no statutory significance in subsequent placement through employment rehabilitation centres and skill centres, they allow people to be presented to industrial rehabilitation with a higher chance of success than if they are presented from the hospital or home without such preparation. In addition, a technical instructor can supervise work that may help to overcome resistance felt by some patients to the sort of craft or skill usually within the compass of occupational therapists. Occupational therapists recognise the problem of giving tasks which are significant and realistic, particularly to patients who have been previously employed on a technical or clerical basis, but may not have the industrial expertise. The skills of a rehabilitation technical instructor, and the workshop facilities that he should have at his disposal, may make a significant contribution to overcoming this problem. At the Swiss Workers' Rehabilitation Unit at Bellikon near Berne the facilities in the workshops are unparalleled; if such munificence is unrepeatable in most places, the principle that goes with it is not.

## VOLUNTARY ORGANISATIONS

There are literally hundreds of organisations that may be involved in the rehabilitation process in different parts of the country. Some will act at the hospital level, such as the League of Friends which is often able to provide such financial support or bits of apparatus which seem not to be forthcoming from the hospital service itself — page-turners, reading aids and so forth. It is also possible that these items may be provided through the Red Cross, and this organisation also has fleets of loan wheelchairs and therefore in emergency may be called on to supplement the provision of appliances. (See also Chapter 12, Future Developments, and the Appendix.)

## THE TEAM APPROACH TO ASSESSMENT
## AND MANAGEMENT

Unfortunately modern management is spewing up a lot of new jargon, the 'team approach' being one such term. This is not to decry the value of the approach itself, but simply to regret the appearance of another bit of misunderstandable jargon. Although details of assessments in each department will be given in the respective chapters, the principle both at Rivermead and at Chessington and at many other rehabilitation centres is that assessment of ability will take place during the first two or three weeks of the patient's stay there on the basis that any shorter period will not allow a period for settling in and that without such a period the original assessments become meaningless. Often the transfer from a hospital where there has been a very protected environment to a rehabilitation centre seems to be accompanied by a regression in performance. Ideally, when members of the team can see the abilities of the patient before they arrive and assess them in the hospital, then this may be discounted or perhaps better clarified in the future. But for the present such knowledge is rare, therefore information is gathered slowly over three weeks and at the end of this time a case conference is held and a formal treatment programme which will hopefully be within the patient's compass is devised. In a rehabilitation centre with 30 or 40 patients it is obviously unrealistic to try to do justice to them all at one conference: some units take new arrivals and assess them in detail and then review, either at special request or at set times, two or three of the patients each week in the future. Other units with perhaps a smaller load of severely brain-damaged patients will attempt to make a full review of the progress of each patient each week, but if so then it has necessarily to be briefer.

## Preparation for discharge

The practice at Rivermead had been to hold a special meeting some weeks prior to discharge when it was felt that progress had slowed to the point where being at the rehabilitation centre had lost its value, and to this meeting were invited not only the therapists concerned but the relatives and representatives of the community health workers and the social workers from the area to which the patient was being discharged. Chessington undertook a similar liaison but because of the distances involved, most patients coming from many hundreds of miles away, it often proved impossible to produce all the relevant parties at a given meeting, so discussion tended to be done rather more by post and over rather a longer period. Obviously the procedure will vary with the catchment area of any individual rehabilitation centre. Whichever method is used, the reintegration of the handicapped person into the community has to be done with great care and gentleness, and when the time appears right then it is reasonable to try to send the patient home either for a day, a weekend or half a week. There is merit in the first introduction to home taking place during the week since if this happens then support services are readily available or readmission can be arranged more easily than at the weekend.

## Allocation of programme time

Details of the amount of hours spent in each department, and the specific tasks that are being set, are usually thrashed out at separate meetings attended by only the therapists concerned, and this also is likely to be a highly effective and practical method of making the system work, though some tact has to be used in order to convince the doctor that he or she does not have to be present at this meeting!

## SETTING UP A NEW
## REHABILITATION CENTRE

Much of what has been said about the question of realistic goal setting for individual patients can be said with equal force to apply to the units themselves. The setting up of a rehabilitation centre is likely to be a costly exercise and its role needs to be clearly stated. There is usually conflict, not only as to who will be responsible for it medically (i.e. the neurosurgeons, orthopaedic surgeons or rehabilitationists), but also as to the role that it should fulfil. Most rehabilitation centres tend to specialise, and the sensible method of setting one up would be to find the problem areas that exist within the existing hospital structure. When, as in the services, the problem is the combination of orthopaedically and neurologically damaged adults, then the way the unit develops is reasonably clear, but in other areas the staff who are responsible for the treatment of stroke may feel that rehabilitation has nothing to offer and will therefore not send patients except to move them from the ward as soon as possible. Yet, if they are not fit to go home, a rehabilitation centre is a cheap way of providing alternative accommodation, and more appropriate to the needs of the patient.

To be of practical value, admission to a rehabilitation unit from the accident and emergency service, or from acute wards, should not be delayed. An ideal situation obtains where the rehabilitation consultant, or members of his team, can visit the hospital where the majority of patients are likely to come from, so that admissions can be arranged in advance.

The facility to offer prompt admission means that for part of the time the unit has to survive criticism for having some spare capacity, or to have some other method of occupying vacant places at a rehabilitation centre which can be cut back at times when admissions are intense. Quite often these times of high admissions can be predicted. There are more likely to be sporting accidents at the beginning of the football season, and road accidents increase during the winter months. Allowing for this spare capacity, however, seems outside the wit of man: wards which are not consistently filled or for which there is not a prolonged waiting list are continually under threat of closure.

If it is important for the rehabilitation consultant to visit the wards from whence his patients come, it is equally important that the accident surgeons maintain liaison with the rehabilitation centre. If the two units are geographically close this requires little effort other than that of goodwill, but if there is a geographical separation then some strategy must be developed whereby there is regular contact between the referring surgeon and the rehabilitation team. If this cannot be achieved, then a penalty will be paid in poor communication.

An example of a civilian rehabilitation centre, linked with a single accident and emergency service, is Rivermead Rehabilitation Centre in Oxford. This is an inpatient unit with 46 beds, of which 30 are fully staffed for 24-hour nursing, and the other 16 are in the nature of hostel accommodation, though having some nursing cover. This unit is orientated to aspects of medical as well as surgical rehabilitation.

There is a large physiotherapy department and gymnasium. Occupational therapy includes workshop, office and clerical departments which allow a wide range of aptitudes to be tested or retrained. It shares with all medical rehabilitation units the impossibility of providing a total range of work assessment; nevertheless, sessions of woodwork, light engineering and office work are possible, and these are complemented by the use of other facilities in and around Oxford. Oxford University and local manufacturers also help in the retraining of patients. The presence of clinical psychologists, speech therapists and psychiatrists on the staff, and the establishment on site of a large social work department, means that the unit can offer many facilities for handicapped patients, and that resettlement can be undertaken at the same time as continuing medical treatment. Because two of the wards have full-time nursing it means that patients can be admitted from hospital earlier than is possible in many rehabilitation centres.

Other patterns of rehabilitation services have been developed. They may either have taken place because of geographical accident or have been developed by surgeons who have had a specific interest in one condition, or again set up specifically by far-sighted managements. No list is likely to be comprehensive, but the rehabilitation centre associated with the Government Training Centre at Garston Manor is one pioneering venture. Campden Road Rehabilitation Centre offers a comprehensive service to those patients for whom it was specifically designed. The author's personal experience would suggest that a mixed centre probably provides the most effective rehabilitation rather than one which is totally specialised to caring for one particular handicap.

## JARGON

The definition of jargon is 'language that is hard to understand because it is full of special words known only to members of a certain group'. Unfortunately, all the medical and paramedical professions are guilty of using jargon, frequently unwittingly, in their day-to-day dealings within the discipline. This often makes it difficult for members of other disciplines, relatives and patients to understand what is going on. Three examples will suffice. 'Behaviour' has a general meaning which we can all understand, but the term has been defined quite precisely by psychologists to whom the meaning is much more restricted and which they now use in a separate way. The same discipline has produced a new meaning for 'generalisation'; most people interpret it as 'a broad sweeping statement', whereas the psychologists are referring to the carryover of an idea from a specific situation into ones that penetrate more deeply into everyday life. Finally, 'client', as defined by the same dictionary, means either 'one who (a) pays a professional person, especially a lawyer, for help and advice' or (b) 'gets help or advice from any of the Government's social services' (for nothing, sic !).

All the contributors to the book have made an effort to reduce or explain their own particular jargon.

# 3

# Anatomy and pathology

## INTRODUCTION

Although prehistoric skulls have shown evidence of healed fracture, it was not until about 1700BC that the first descriptions of head injury were recorded by the Egyptians in what is now known as the Edwin Smith Papyrus. Bleeding from the nose or ears with shudderings (convulsions) are described, together with eye deformity (deviation), shuffling gait and one who does not release the shoulder fork (hemiplegic) posture of the arm. The first record of the change in personality and mental state was not made until 1848, when Phineas Gage, a capable foreman, was placing dynamite down a deep hole with a tamping rod, and suddenly the latter was blown through his jaw, his eye and out through the top of his head. Dr Harlow, to whose surgery he walked, managed to extract the rod, and 20 years later obtained the skull (Fig. 3.1). He wrote the following description in 1848:

... General appearance good: stands quite erect, with his head inclined slightly towards the right side: his gait in walking is steady: his movements rapid, and easily executed ... His physical health is good, and I am inclined to say that he has recovered. Has no pain in head, but says it has a queer feeling which he is not able to describe. Applied for his situation as foreman, but is undecided whether to work or travel. His contractors, who regarded him as the most efficient and capable foreman in their employ previous to his injury, considered the change in his mind so marked that they could not give him his place again. The equilibrium or balance, so to speak, between his intellectual faculties and animal propensities, seems to have been destroyed. He is fitful, irreverent, indulging at times in the grossest profanity (which was not previously his custom), manifesting but little deference for his fellows, impatient of restraint or advice when it conflicts with his desires, at times pertinaciously obstinate yet capricious and vacillating, devising

27

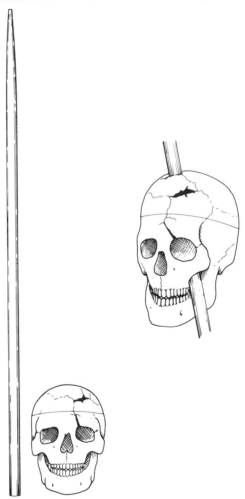

**Fig. 3.1**  Phineas Gage.

many plans of future operation, which are no sooner arranged than they are abandoned in turn for others appearing more feasible. A child in his intellectual capacity and manifestations, he has the animal passions of a strongman. Previous to his injury, though untrained in the schools, he possessed a well-balanced mind, and was looked upon by those who knew him as a shrewd, smart business man, very energetic and persistent in executing all his plans of operation. In this regard his mind was radically changed, so decidedly that his friends and acquaintances said he was 'no longer Gage'. (J. M. Harlow, 1868.)

## ANATOMY OF THE SKULL AND BRAIN

### Macroscopic and microscopic anatomy

Essentially the skull is a rigid, rounded box of bone, with an irregular floor which completely surrounds and protects the soft brain from direct injury. The floor is in three parts, or fossae, the anterior part being shallow above the orbits, the middle one dropping down over the sharp sphenoidal ridge and lying over the inner ear, and the posterior part lying even lower. The skull is lined by a thick, tough, fibrous membrane, the dura mater, which subdivides the skull cavity by thick sheet-like extensions: the falx cerebri which extends vertically from front to back, and the tentorium which lies at right angles separating the occipital lobes from the cerebellum (Fig. 3.2). The tentorium cerebelli has a large gap in its central portion extending anteriorly, through which the mid-brain passes. The most important fact to grasp is the total rigidity of the skull itself, its irregular ridges and indentations in its base, and the equally rigid extensions of the dura.

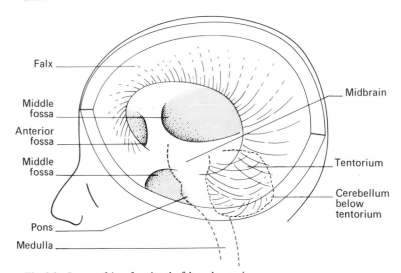

**Fig. 3.2**  Layers of dura forming the falx and tentorium.

The softer but incompressible brain is surrounded by a thin membrane, the pia mater, which is surrounded in turn by a loosely attached, thin, outer membrane, the arachnoid. Between the pia mater and the arachnoid membrane is the subarachnoid space in which run the blood vessels supplying and draining the superficial substance of the brain. Blood from the heart reaches them through arteries which pierce the floor of the skull and dura to provide oxygenated blood to both the deep and superficial structures of the brain. The arteries divide into progressively smaller branches to ramify throughout the whole of the brain. The superficial ones tend to anastomose with each other, but this does not occur in the deep penetrating central branches. Blood is thus distributed through the whole brain and is drained through a venous system back to the heart.

The brain is made up of two cerebral hemispheres linked together by a massive bridge, the corpus callosum. Within these hemispheres, lying more centrally, are the accumulation of nerve cells of the corpus striatum and below them the diencephalon, or between-brain. Immediately behind the latter, the brain stem runs downwards and backwards within the head, passing through the tentorium to the foramen magnum at the base of the skull where it becomes the spinal cord. The whole is bathed by cerebrospinal fluid (CSF) from the choroid plexuses largely in the lateral ventricles inside the brain, and this CSF flows downwards through the third ventricle in the diencephalon and down the brain stem along the aqueduct of Sylvius to the fourth ventricle within the posterior part of the brain. The CSF then passes from inside the ventricular system to the subarachnoid space through three foramina below the tentorium and superior to the cerebellum. From there it travels back over the convexity and across the base of the brain to be drawn finally through little granulations into the main venous sinuses.

The brain consists of firm grey matter which is a concentration of nerve cells and white soft matter which is an intercommunicating fibre system. The grey matter spreads over the convoluted surface forming the cortex and is collected into large, mainly bilateral masses, e.g. the corpus striatum and thalamus, deep within the hemispheres. It continues down the brain stem both in bilateral collections forming the cranial nuclei and as widely scattered nerve cells, many of which are tiny intercalating neurones. The cerebellum is a specialised portion of the brain lying posteriorly to the brain stem beneath the tentorium and is likewise made up of a nuclear cortex and nuclear masses within its substance with intercommunicating white matter. The neurones (the nerve cells) and their processes are supported throughout the brain by a framework of neuroglia (supportive cells). Each individual neurone (see Fig. 3.3) consists of a cell body, a nucleus and one or more processes (the dendrites) which receive impulses and one process (the axon) which propagates the impulses. The white matter consists of axons and neuroglia. There are many different specialised types of neurones (Fig. 3.3) with dendrites of varying density and number and axons of different diameter and length. Some neurones have bipolar axons similar to dorsal root ganglion cells. The longest axons of

NEURONE

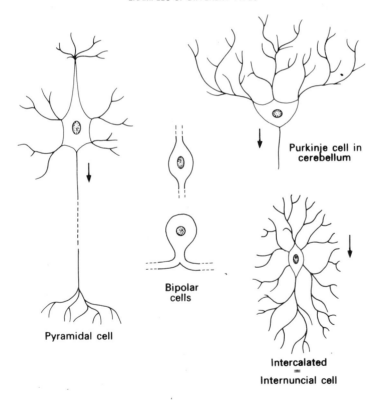

Direction of
impulse

Axon

Myelin
sheath

Nucleus

Dendrites

EXAMPLES OF DIFFERENT TYPES

Purkinje cell in
cerebellum

Bipolar
cells

Pyramidal cell

Intercalated
=
Internuncial cell

**Fig. 3.3**    Drawing of neurone and examples of different neurones.

all are those of the pyramidal cells of the cortex which may extend over one metre in length. Most of the smallest intercalating neurones have processes of microscopic length. All communications between neurones are made chemically at synapses while the nerve impulses are propagated electrically along axons by depolarisation. The anatomical arrangement is much the same whether the neurones are functioning at a subconscious or at a conscious level. The neuroglia (see Fig. 3.4), on the other hand, are of three main types: the astrocytes which are closely related to the blood vessels, the oligodendroglia which lie along the fibres maintaining the myelin, and the microglia which are phagocytic in nature and work as scavengers by rounding up and ingesting any debris or other broken down, unwanted matter.

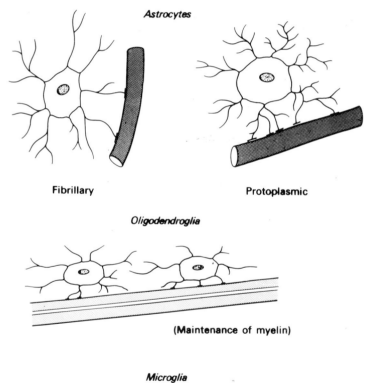

**Astrocytes**

Fibrillary                    Protoplasmic

*Oligodendroglia*

(Maintenance of myelin)

*Microglia*

(Phagocytic) removes debris

**Fig. 3.4**   Neuroglia (supporting cells).

Thus it can be appreciated that the substance of the brain varies in density with relatively firm nuclear masses and cortex, joined by softer fibre tracts and bridges. It will be remembered that the whole lies within a rigid skull, divided by the septa of the dura. In summary, three important points emerge: (i) the rigidity of the skull and septa of the dura; (ii) the relative firmness of neuronal masses and the softness of the fibre tracts and bridges; (iii) widespread ramifications of the vascular tree, both within and surrounding the brain substance.

## PATHOLOGY

**Macroscopic pathology**

It is important to differentiate between open and closed head injury. An open major head wound (i.e. with the dura punctured), as sustained from a bullet, a circular saw or a hatchet, causes localised destruction with relative sparing of the rest of the brain. Closed head injury occurs when the head is free to move and while there is no apparent external wound there may be fracture of the skull. Road traffic accidents have caused an enormous rise in the incidence of closed head injury over the past few years. This type of injury occurs when there is sudden acceleration of the head, e.g. when the car in which the person is sitting is hit from behind; likewise, it occurs in deceleration, with or without twisting, e.g. by the moving head hitting against a stationary object. Common causes of this injury are being thrown from a motorcycle, falling from a roof or children's slide or even, in an older person, falling at home or outdoors. Where the person is thrown about inside a car, a moving head may be hit several times from different directions, so that many lines of stress, twisting and shearing occur.

Concussion and damage is produced much more easily in the head which is free to move (Denny Brown & Russell 1941). Professional boxers and footballers heading the ball minimise concussion by fixing the head in space at the moment of impact. Brain substance is incompressible, like the cerebrospinal fluid in which it floats. Holbourn (1943) studied the effects of a blow on the brain using gelatine models (see Fig. 3.5) and showed that distortion occurred inside with shifting of some parts relative to other parts. He also found that the same areas were damaged constantly in relation to particular directions of the blow to the models. He predicted that this mechanism was responsible for the damage sustained in closed head injury. Pudenz & Sheldon (1946) showed by means of high-speed cinematography in monkeys, in whom part of the skull had been replaced with transparent material, that, if the head was free to move,

SHEAR STRAINS IN GELATIN MODELS

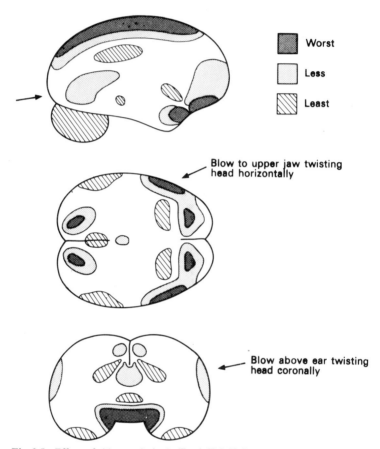

Fig. 3.5   Effects of a blow on the brain (Dr. A.H.S. Holbourn).

the brain twisted and swirled even with weak blows insufficient to
cause concussion. They also observed that the brain did not separate
away from the skull at any time during or immediately after impact as
had previously been believed. Thus it can be understood that during a
blow to a freely moving head the softer more friable structures move
faster (see Fig. 3.5), sliding upon each other according to the direction
of stress or twist. They swirl around the more dense nuclear masses
and may be stretched near the falx or the edge of the tentorium. The
cortex and main nuclear masses are relatively spared at the expense of
white matter where nerve fibres are torn or stretched. Many small
fibres may be broken during twisting and deformation of the brain
stem. Small blood vessels are also torn, throughout the hemispheres,

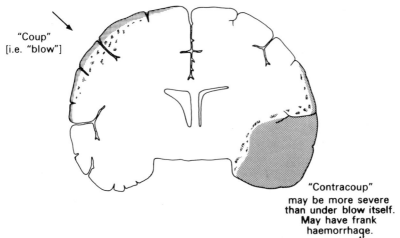

"Coup"
[i.e. "blow"]

"Contracoup"
may be more severe
than under blow itself.
May have frank
haemorrhage.

**Fig. 3.6** 'Coup' and 'contracoup'.

brain stem and cerebellum, causing minute scattered haemorrhages.

After rupture of larger vessels, frank haemorrhage may occur particularly over the frontal and temporal poles. It may also occur in 'coup' and 'contracoup' (see Fig. 3.6), when bruising occurs under the site of a direct blow and on the opposite side of the brain in the line of the blow where the bruising is generally more severe. Overt haemorrhage is not usually as devastating to the person as the scattered shearing of nerve fibres and patchy destruction of the great intercommunicating networks.

The apparently normal appearance of the brain after closed head injury, apart from visible lacerations and haemorrhage, was not realised to be misleading until the middle of the twentieth century. Before this time clinicians and pathologists had been content to diagnose injury to the brain in the following ways:

1. 'If blood comes from the nostrils, the ears and the neck be stiff [after head injury] — a condition not to be treated.' (Edwin Smith Papyrus.)

2. Concussion
   Unconsciousness occurs with either subsequent recovery, with no apparent neurological signs, or death with a brain that appears normal at autopsy.

3. Extradural haemorrhage
   This results from rupture of the middle meningeal artery, e.g. in the case of a footballer who is rendered unconscious by a blow to the head, quickly recovers and finishes the game, only to become unconscious later with a developing hemiplegia. Evacuation of the clot and subsequent repair leads to full recovery.

4. Subdural haemorrhage
   Unconsciousness persists from the start, and only incomplete recovery is likely to follow removal of the clot from beneath the dura.
5. 'Coup' and 'contracoup'

## PATHOLOGY

**Microscopic pathology**
Strich (1956, 1961) examined brains from people who had suffered from closed head injury and survived for periods of 48 hours up to two years. On first examination, the brains looked almost normal, though many had slight haemorrhages in the corpus callosum and the superior cerebellar peduncle. Brains of a few patients with longer survival showed small scattered yellow cysts (evidence of old haemorrhage with healing) and most of these brains had some dilatation of the ventricular system. On microscopy with new techniques at 48 hours, Strich saw many ruptured nerve fibres scattered through the brain with 'retraction balls' due to the extrusion of axoplasm from each end of broken nerve fibre. Present were many large phagocytic cells (rounded-up microglia) containing fat granules from the simultaneous disruption and ensuing breakdown of the fatty myelin sheaths surrounding the fibres. These fibres appeared to have been interrupted along particular lines of stress so that the swollen axons and retraction balls looked like shoals of fish.

Nerve fibres degenerate when separated from the parent cell body or when the latter dies. This degeneration leads to withering of the tracts of the affected nerve fibres: e.g. the pyramidal tract, which is frequently involved, may wither along its entire length extending right down the spinal cord. Widespread degeneration of the nerve fibre tracts is accompanied by demyelination. The myelin is replaced by large phagocytic cells packed with fat granules.

Oppenheimer (1968), using other techniques, has also demonstrated the presence of diffuse microscopic lesions even in the brains of patients who have survived less than a day. Tiny microglial reactions, leading to microglial scars, form in response to tearing or stretching of nerve fibres without haemorrhage or to tiny capillary haemorrhages. Reactive astrocytes start to appear after three weeks around the larger collections of microglia.

## APPLIED ANATOMY

While certain parts of the brain are principally responsible for particular functions, it normally performs as a whole. After brain damage the clinical deficits result not only from a loss of localised brain function but also from the functioning of those parts of the brain which have been preserved, either wholly or in part, and which are now performing without the normal inhibitions and interactions from higher and other centres. Patchy continuity of the interconnecting pathways may exist and recent experimental work has shown that small outgrowths from existing dendrites of nerve cells may occur to form new connections. Although new cells cannot be formed to replace dead ones, the surviving brain has a remarkable capacity to take over lost functions to some extent. This knowledge has been acquired by careful observation of patients with good pathological correlation, and by a great deal of detailed experimental work over the past 200 years.

Each half of the brain controls the opposite half of the body in response to the reception of sensory input, by suppressing the unwanted encoded material which first passes to both halves of the brain. The central sulcus separates each cerebral hemisphere (Fig. 3.7) roughly into an anterior motor expressive portion, the frontal lobes, and the posterior receptive part, the parietal, occipital and

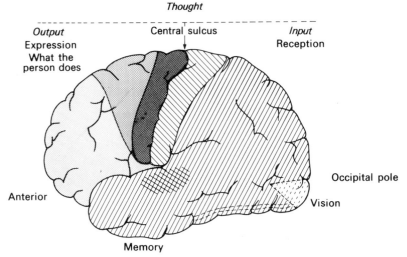

**Fig. 3.7** Functions common to both hemispheres.

temporal lobes, which receive the primary sensations of touch and proprioception, temperature and pain, vision and hearing and smell respectively. The frontal lobes anteriorly are mainly concerned with initiative, foresight, judgement and the formulation of ideas resulting directly from the sensory input which has already been encoded in the light of previous experience and knowledge. Immediately anterior to the central sulcus, the precentral gyrus superimposes fine skilled movements, particularly those of the face and hands of the opposite side, on to the generalised gross movements driven from much lower centres and already modulated to smoothness and aimed in the correct direction through the cerebellar and extrapyramidal systems. The latter project from the frontal cortex anterior to the precentral gyrus. In the dominant precentral gyrus itself, the mouth parts and hands are particularly well represented, and are responsible for the intricate, very rapid and finely coordinated movements required for speech and manual dexterity.

## Perception
Perception of sensation requires several stages. The first stage is the ability of the body to convert an external physical stimulus into a form which the nervous system can handle (transduction). For example, light, sound, smell are all transduced by the peripheral sense organs into nerve impulses that are capable of being transmitted to the brain. The brain itself is capable of registering this information, of comparing it with past experience, and is then able to 'perceive' only that which is needful. Otherwise the potential input that is available from the environment could swamp a relevant stimulus. This is sometimes clinically apparent after brain damage.

The parietal lobe is primarily responsible for the interpretation of the sensations of touch, pain, temperature, and proprioception, the occipital lobe for vision and the temporal lobe for smell, balance, hearing, a major part of memory and sexual drive.

### Touch, pain and temperature
When the sensations of touch, pain and temperature reach the parietal lobe cortex and particularly the post-central gyrus, then the actual nature of the sensation comes into a conscious level. The parietal cortex is responsible for fine discrimination of different degrees of temperature, or of pain, or of the nature of pain, and in particular the discrimination of two points in space. If two or more separate points in space can be appreciated separately, then objects touching the skin, particularly in the hands, can be recognised both for size, shape, weight, texture and nature.

For example, if minimal loss of touch is present in the hand, it is possible for a patient to recognise a large, heavy, well-known object, e.g. a comb, by touch, but he is quite unable to observe the difference between velvet and sandpaper or between a screw and a nail. This loss of the power of discrimination (astereognosis) is always associated with defective two-point discrimination. If the parietal area is still partially preserved it is possible that the ordinary fine tests of discrimination on the opposite side of the body are normal, but that the sensory stimuli cannot be felt there when both sides of the body are stimulated simultaneously with equal stimuli. The latter effect is known as an inattention for sensation. It can thus be understood that, if partial interruption of the main fine discriminatory sensory pathway has occurred at a lower level, defective sensory input reaches the cortex, in which case the brain receives insufficient information at a high level to be able to 'compute' how to move that side of the body appropriately (one form of apraxia).

*Vision*
The visual cortex lies at the occipital pole of the brain and along the calcarine fissure on the medial aspect of each occipital lobe. It receives impulses along the primary visual system. The retina of each eye receives the visual input from the focused optical images of the environment: the fibres from the nasal half of the retina of each eye decussate, travelling back to the lateral geniculate body on the opposite side (Fig. 3.8). The fibres arising from each temporal half of the retina travel to the lateral geniculate body without decussation on the ipsilateral side. The optic radiations arise from the lateral geniculate body on each side and travel first of all forward and upward and laterally, and finally backwards through the substance of each cerebral hemisphere to reach the visual cortex. Thus, the cortex on each side receives input from the opposite visual half field. As the visual system is a direct point to point anatomical system, interruption of function at any particular level can be recognised accurately from the clinical deficit. This is well described in all neurological textbooks.

*Hearing, balance, smell, sexual drive and memory*
The temporal lobes subserve the senses of hearing, balance, smell and a major part of memory. The dominant temporal lobe is principally responsible for verbal memory whereas non-verbal memory is processed mainly by the non-dominant temporal lobe. Hearing and balance are represented in the temporal lobe on either side, so auditory understanding is not lost until the auditory cortex is destroyed bilaterally. However, many devastating defects occur in auditory understanding and in high level comprehension as the result of partial damage of the auditory cortex or of its immediate connections.

*Sexual drive*
Sexual drive may also be altered from temporal lobe deficits which, though commonly associated with impotence or failure to maintain a

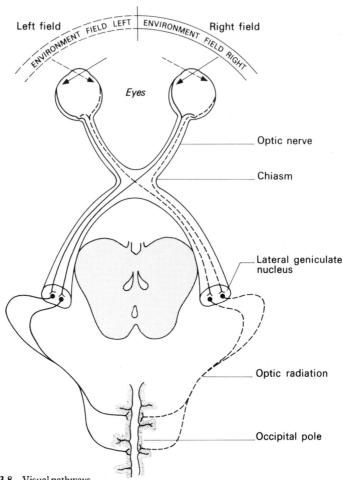

**Fig. 3.8** Visual pathways.

good erection, may also be associated with increased libido and sexual drive.

### Smell
In head injury, loss or reduction of smell is generally the result of destruction of the fibres as they pass back from the nose into the anterior part of the brain and not from lesions of the receptive region in the temporal lobes. This condition occurs commonly in fractures of the base of the skull and is usually permanent.

The large area joining the parietal, occipital and temporal lobes and their interconnections is responsible for the integration of the different forms of sensation, leading to the understanding of sensory input: that which is seen and heard, in particular the understanding of symbols as in spoken language and the written word. Without comprehension of language or the significance of visual input, of proprioception or feeling, the patient loses the ability to function normally in relation to his environment.

## Speech

In early life speech is represented on both sides of the brain, but, as the child develops, one cerebral hemisphere becomes dominant and speech develops to a high degree in that hemisphere. This is generally the dominant left hemisphere in a right-handed person. In the adult, the dominant hemisphere has the principal responsibility for language, i.e. comprehension of spoken or written language, and the execution of speech and writing, together with verbal memory (Fig. 3.9). Frequently mathematical calculation and orientation between left and right are also located there. Comprehension of speech is a function of the dominant temporoparieto-occipital cortex and this is linked by interconnecting neurones with the anterior part of the frontal lobe, where further processing leads to sequencing of ideas and

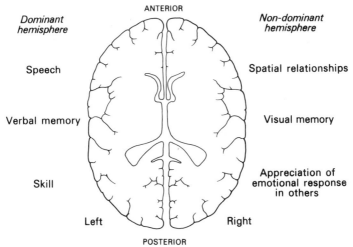

Fig. 3.9 Individual functions of cerebral hemispheres.

language, and thereby to expression, either by speaking, writing or with other skilled movements (see Chapter 4).

## Visual memory and spatial relationships

The non-dominant hemisphere (i.e. the right hemisphere in a right-handed person) is concerned particularly with visual memory and spatial relationships. These include the awareness of body image and orientation in space, and also relationships between the different parts of the body in space and to each other (Fig. 3.9). The relative distances of objects, both stationary and moving in the environment, together with the shapes and recognition of objects and faces in the light of previous experience, i.e. visual memory, are also functions of the non-dominant hemisphere. In addition the latter is believed to be responsible for the virtually subconscious appreciation of the emotional response of other people or animals, and probably plays a large part in the appreciation and understanding of music.

**Subconscious control**
Deep within the hemispheres and rostral to the mid-brain lie the great nuclear masses of the extrapyramidal system (corpus striatum) and thalami. They subserve posture and movement in response to subconscious stimuli from somatic sensory, proprioceptive, visual, vestibular and cerebellar input. The extrapyramidal system has large cortical radiations to and from the frontal lobe, while the thalamus has large cortical projections to both frontal and parietal lobes.

The thalami are not only sensory but also play a large part in the motor integration through the extrapyramidal system. Beneath the thalami lies the hypothalamus, which controls the autonomic nervous system — the parasympathetic and sympathetic innervation of the opposite side of the body, and responsible for maintaining body temperature, water balance, carbohydrate and fat metabolism and gonadal activity (Fig. 3.10).

Within the mid-brain and upper brain stem, the reticular activating system extends dorsally and is responsible for controlling sleep and wakefulness. The upper brain stem is particularly liable to be damaged in any rotational head injury, and it may also be compressed or squashed downwards against the rigid tentorium. It is believed that concussion arises primarily from damage to this region. Akinetic mutism is thought to be related to the abnormal functioning of the reticular activating system.

## THE BRAIN STEM

*The brain stem*, which can be subdivided into the mid-brain, pons and medulla, contains the nuclei of the IIIrd to XIIth cranial nerves, details of which can be found in any standard textbook of anatomy. However, the IIIrd, IVth and VIth nerves are of particular interest, as they subserve eye movement and control the individual eye muscles.

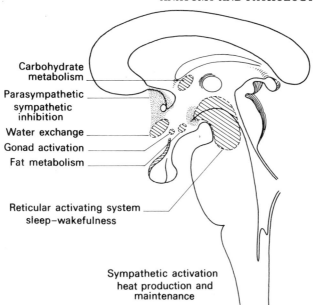

Carbohydrate
metabolism

Parasympathetic
sympathetic
inhibition

Water exchange

Gonad activation

Fat metabolism

Reticular activating system
sleep-wakefulness

Sympathetic activation
heat production and
maintenance

**Fig. 3.10**   Hypothalamic nuclei and reticular activating system.

These bilateral nuclei are joined together by the medial longitudinal fasciculus (Fig. 3.11), which not only interconnects the nuclei so that the eyes normally remain parallel when moving (conjugate gaze), but also relays impulses to them from the semicircular canals via the vestibular nuclei and from proprioceptive impulses from the neck muscles. Control of speed and smoothness of these eye movements is carried out by the cerebellum, thalami and extrapyramidal systems, while the actual direction of lateral gaze is controlled voluntarily from the frontal cortex through a lower gaze centre. The pathways for upgaze and downgaze pass through the quadrigeminal body on the posterior aspect of the mid-brain. The mid-brain and upper pons, which contain these eye nuclei, together with the superior cerebellar peduncle (going to the thalamus) are again particularly susceptible to the twisting, swirling, stretching and compression against the tentorium that can follow a blow to the unrestrained skull. Likewise, if any increase of intracranial content from bleeding or later from brain oedema secondary to anoxia causes a downward pressure and herniation of forebrain tissue through the rigid tentorial opening (coning), then vital neurones controlling eye movements and balance are at considerable risk of compression or destruction, in addition to any local tearing of blood vessels. It is therefore not surprising that abnormal eye signs are usually present after severe head injury. If a nucleus or its nerve to an eye muscle is compressed or destroyed, then

MEDIAL LONGITUDINAL FASCICULUS

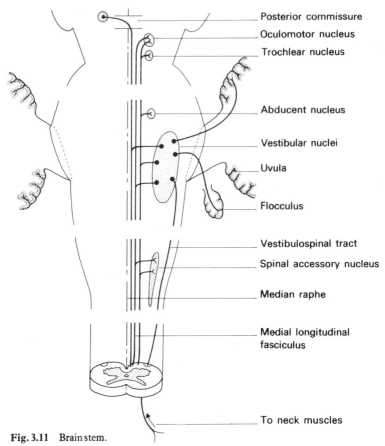

Fig. 3.11   Brain stem.

total paralysis of that movement ensues. The IIIrd nerve (oculomotor) nucleus contains sections which supply different eye muscles, together with other separated central subnuclei supplying the parasympathetic control of construction of the pupil. The IIIrd nerve is particularly liable to be damaged at its point of emergence from the brain stem and complete severance or compression causes immediate fixed dilatation of the pupil. During coning, however, the pressure above the tentorium may vary, so that a previously normal constricted pupil may be seen to dilate and constrict, perhaps several times before finally dilating permanently and being no longer capable of reacting to light. This is why observation of the pupil after any form of head injury or intracranial operation is so important, as it monitors the state of intracranial pressure above the tentorium.

The pons and medulla contain the nuclei for the remaining cranial nerves and many individual interconnecting nuclei, some of which are sensory, receiving impulses from the cerebellum and spinal cord, and some of which are motor, receiving impulses from all levels from the cortex downwards. There are also many other interconnecting neurones. The main vestibular pathways cross the pons to the opposite side on their way to the thalamus and corpus striatum. Lower down the cardiovascular and respiratory vital centres are situated within the dorsal part of the medulla, while anteriorly the olives, consisting of proprioceptive relay cells between the spinal cord and cerebellum, bulge from the surface. The medulla is also greatly at risk during coning since it can be forced downwards through the foramen magnum, causing severe compression of its substance so that blood can no longer circulate to the vital centres. These cease to function causing cardiac arrest, circulatory and respiratory failure, Slowing of the pulse with a rising blood pressure are other indications of rising intracranial pressure.

During the actual impact of closed head injury, physical damage can be done at one or many points within the substance of the brain. The clinical state immediately afterwards reflects major areas of neuronal and fibre damage, but the effects of secondary anoxia with subsequent cerebral oedema and coning can develop with terrifying rapidity if the respiratory and cardiovascular centres do not start functioning within a very few minutes. If they recover but the airway is not clear because the patient is lying supine or has inhaled vomit or had a crushed chest or multiple injuries, with or without profuse loss of blood, anoxia of the brain still supervenes. This rapidly causes oedema of the brain producing further anoxia adding further great damage, particularly to the nerve cells of the cortex of both the cerebral hemispheres and cerebellum to that already done in the initial injury. It is thus clear that it is essential to prevent the onset of anoxia by maintaining a clear airway and preventing haemorrhage as far as possible in head injured patients, from the moment of impact. Pneumonia at a later stage must be prevented if possible to reduce the risk of further anoxic damage to the brain.

**Clinical deficits**
An infinite variety of clinical deficits can be seen after acute closed head injury. All injuries affect the function of the mind from the moment of impact (see Chapter 9). However, certain combinations of physical defects occur relatively so frequently together that they are worth separate consideration.

1. The spastic diplegia from the bilateral loss of the pyramidal tracts at any level within the brain
   This is generally more severe on one side and is associated with loss of movement and of volitional control of the limbs with difficulty in speech and swallowing. The spasticity may become very great and may be associated with extra-pyramidal rigidity or dystonic posture of part or whole of the body.

2. Hemiplegia with cerebellar ataxia on the opposite side
   This arises from involvement of the pyramidal tract on one side with lesions in the superior cerebellar peduncle.

3. Hemiplegia which may be motor and/or sensory with or without visual defect

4. Eye signs
   a. Nystagmus
   Nystagmus or ataxia of eye movement, is seen in lesions of the cerebellum and/or its central connections. Nystagmus on lateral gaze is commonly associated with lesions in the cerebellar hemispheres, while vertical nystagmus, or nystagmus with the gaze directed straight ahead, is generally associated with damage to the more central connections within the brain stem. If minimal, nystagmus may only be recognised as jerky rather than smooth movements, as the eyes turn from side to side.
   b. Loss of conjugate gaze
   At rest this is usually manifest by squints of varying degree. When the eyes look to one side, the leading eye moves quicker than the following eye, which, as soon as the leading eye fixes on a new object, moves over, perhaps even overshooting the line of parallel gaze before settling back again, often to some divergence. This is seen in lesions within the upper brain stem affecting the medial longitudinal fasciculus with or without damage to its connections with the quadrigeminal plate and the gaze centre.
   c. Paralysis of eye muscles
   In head injury, the paralysis generally results from compression, distortion or fracture of the IIIrd and VIth cranial nerves, less commonly of the IVth. When any muscles is separated from its nerve, total paralysis ensures. Total paralysis of the IIIrd nerve causes complete closure of the eyelid. The eye itself cannot be moved up, medially or down, and the pupil is widely dilated and fixed. Paralysis of the VIth nerve causes loss of lateral movement. Paralysis of the IVth nerve is rarely seen and the eye is then unable to move down and in. If one group of muscles only is paralysed the

action of the other muscles which are still innervated will tend to pull the eye towards those active muscles.

d. The pupils

The muscles of the pupils are controlled by the parasympathetic and sympathetic nerve supply. The parasympathetic travels with the IIIrd nerve and when the latter ceases to function for any reason then the pupils are affected, in addition to paralysis of certain eye muscles. The pupil is widely dilated and does not react to light, either directly or consensually, nor to accommodation. The parasympathetic subnuclei within the IIIrd nerve nucleus are midline and single whereas those IIIrd nerve nuclei innervating the eye muscles are bilaterally represented. The sympathetic nerve supply arises from the sympathetic chain of ganglia in the neck and travels with the carotid and then the ophthalmic artery to the eye. The sympathetic nerve, when stimulated, causes dilatation of the pupil, and if paralysed, the pupil becomes very small and unreactive, provided the parasympathetic nerve supply is intact. The sympathetic supply of the pupil is controlled from the hypothalamus through fibres running in the brain stem and spinal cord down to the level of the first thoracic segment from which they emerge to reach the sympathetic ganglia. Pupillary abnormalities may result from either central or peripheral interruption of these pathways.

e. Blindness — partial or complete

This may occur in interruption of the primary visual pathway at any point between the optic nerve within the orbit to the visual cortex at the occipital pole. Thus there may be complete loss of vision from severance of the optic nerve or chiasm or from bilateral destruction of the occipital poles. Hemianopia or quadrantanopia generally result from destruction within the optic tract or the optic radiations. Macular sparing, that is sparing of central vision, results when there is almost complete destruction of the optic radiation but with preservation of the occipital pole and some macular fibres. Visual loss may also be patchy in head injury, or be due to a combination of several superimposed areas of destruction.

f. Colour vision

Loss, or incomplete loss, of colour vision is usually due to stretching or ischaemia of the optic nerve especially the macular fibres which are more susceptible than those arising more peripherally in the retina. Vision may also be lost with destruction in the poster-inferior part of the junction between the temporal and occipital lobes. This loss may not necessarily be complete and there may be improvement with time, during which defective matching of different shades of the same colour may be found. Whether recovery is total or incomplete, depends on the extent of the original damage.

*Perceptual disorders.* The interpretation and integration of the significance and meaning of the primary visual input is a function of the large area of cerebral cortex between the temporoparietal and occipital lobes. It has been shown in experimental animals that there are many relays of cells extending forwards in the cortex of this area, which are responsible for progressive encoding of the original input. A disorder of perception is said to be present when a patient in whom sight is preserved is no longer able to understand that which he can see, neither can he interpret the spatial relationships between objects around him nor of his own position in his environment. This can take many forms in varying degrees, but it is frequently impossible for the patient to appreciate that he is not perceiving correctly. Some patients are unable to find their way about. Others cannot recognise faces of people they know well. There is frequently loss of visual memory, for although it is unlikely that the cortical cells themselves will be much damaged during closed head injury, the underlying fibres, dendrites and axons are greatly at risk from the sliding of the various layers upon each other. Likewise, the corpus callosum, which is very valuable at the time of injury, from distortion and stretching, may be damaged in many areas leading to loss of direct communication between the two hemispheres which can no longer work together in the interpretation of the visual input. Lesions in these areas of the white matter of the cerebral hemispheres and corpus callosum are thought to be responsible for the so-called 'disconnection syndromes'.


APRAXIA/DYSPRAXIA

Apraxia is the total inability in a patient to produce volitional movement specially to order, when he can perform the same movement involuntarily, showing that the actual mechanism for the movement is present, e.g. he cannot protrude tongue to command but can lick a stamp and stick it on an envelope. It can arise from faulty sensory input, from lack of being able to form the correct ideas in the correct sequence to carry out a movement, and finally in the actual conversion of the idea to the movement itself. Apraxia can arise from lesions on either side of the brain, either posteriorly or anteriorly, or in the corpus callosum, and is thought to be due to a lack of continuity in the normal pathways for initiating volitional movement.

*Case example*

Mr N has a mild bilateral hemiplegia following a moderate head injury, during which he also sustained a fractured right femur. The latter injury was slow to heal and the femur was eventually pinned. After months of intensive rehabilitation, the patient was still unable to form the idea of how to walk well with his operated leg. He was able to walk with a good normal swing when in parallel bars, being encouraged verbally and by mime, but he relapsed at once when reinforcement was withdrawn. The fundamental difficulty here was the inability to form the idea of how to walk, that is, apraxia for walking. Without the recognition of the presence of apraxia, by the rehabilitation team, and by the understanding of the patient's relatives and friends, walking could not be achieved.

## SUMMARY

The main features of closed head injury are:

1. The rigidity of the skull and septa of the dura. The incompressibility of the brain and CSF. Unrestrained movement of the head at the time of injury

2. Primary damage, at the time of head injury
   a. Swirling and slipping of layers of connecting white matter with shearing of nerve fibres
   b. Shearing of minute blood vessels causing scattered minute haemorrhages
   c. Haemorrhage, contusion, lacerations especially at poles, particularly frontal and temporal, both 'coup' and 'contracoup'
   d. Destruction of neurones by (a), (b) and (c)

3. Secondary damage superimposed due to
   a. Anoxia from faulty airway, chest injuries
   b. Cerebral oedema, from anoxia, causing a vicious circle of further oedema and anoxia leading to increased intracranial tension and coning
   c. Failure of circulation and respiration aggravating (a) and (b)
   d. Cerebral anaemia from loss of blood elsewhere in body

4. After prolonged survival
   Widespread degeneration of nerve fibres in white matter and long tracts. Replacement of the latter with diffuse microglial proliferation, microglial clusters, diffuse increase of astrocytes, fat-containing cells.

5. Degree of recovery depends on: (i) extent of original damage; (ii) extent of secondary damage due to anoxia and anaemia; (iii) plasticity and ability of the brain to develop alternative circuits, which decrease with advancing age, underlying disease, alcoholism,

and after repeated injuries to the head; (iv) early mental and physical stimulation and active rehabilitation are believed to promote greater eventual recovery.

## REFERENCES

Denny Brown D, Russell W R 1941 Journal of Physiology 99: 153

Holbourn A H S 1943 Lancet ii: 438

Oppenheimer D R 1968 Journal of Neurology, Neurosurgery and Psychiatry 31: 229-306

Pudenz R H, Sheldon C H 1946 Journal of Neurosurgery 3: 487

Rowbotham G F 1945 Acute Injuries to the Head, 2nd edn. E & S Livingstone, Edinburgh

Strich S J 1956 Journal of Neurology, Neurosurgery and Psychiatry 19: 163-185

Strich S J 1961 Lancet ii: 443-448

# 4

# Speech therapy

## INTRODUCTION

Talking is important for everyone and can be taken for granted until something goes wrong. There are very few activities which do not involve verbal communication, whether spoken or written: for example, conversation with neighbours, listening to the radio, or television, shopping, reading road signs, departure boards and maps, attending an interview or receiving instructions at work. Without the ability to understand and talk and to a lesser degree to read and write, the quality of life is much poorer. A second equally important and closely related factor on which normal living depends is the ability to remember. It is impossible to hold a conversation unless the preceding sentence can be remembered, and there is no point in looking up the time of trains unless the information is retained. The speech therapist's role in rehabilitation of the brain-damaged patient is not only to deal with communication difficulties, both in speech and language, but also with defects in memory, since memory is an integral part of communication.

## NORMAL LANGUAGE

The basic structure of normal language must be considered before treating patients with abnormal language. Therefore, the pathways involved in understanding and talking will be considered first, then the disabilities which sometimes follow a head injury, and finally aspects of general management.

### Normal communication

The pathways of normal communication can be illustrated as a circuit with input and output channels as well as a store. (See Fig. 4.1.)

### Comprehension of spoken language

*Hearing*
Hearing is the ability to receive sound waves through the ear. This is of course essential for understanding speech.

**The basic structure of normal spoken language**

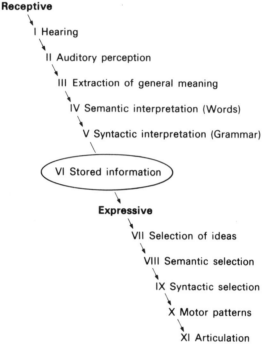

**Receptive**

I Hearing

II Auditory perception

III Extraction of general meaning

IV Semantic interpretation (Words)

V Syntactic interpretation (Grammar)

VI Stored information

**Expressive**

VII Selection of ideas

VIII Semantic selection

IX Syntactic selection

X Motor patterns

XI Articulation

Fig. 4.1

*Auditory perception*
This is the ability to recognise that speech sounds are potentially meaningful and discriminate these from other background sounds.

*Extraction of general meaning*
Before processing semantics and syntax, a large part of comprehension relies on appreciating accompanying factors, e.g. facial expression, gesture and tone of voice.

*Semantic interpretation*
The meaning of each individual word in a sentence has to be understood. Most words are unambiguous but some sound the same, and the difference can only be appreciated from the context, e.g. bough/bow, sale/sail.

*Syntactic interpretation*
This is the ability to understand grammatical constructions and the order of words. The order can alter the meaning of a sentence, e.g. 'The boy ran past the stream' has a completely different meaning from 'The stream ran past the boy'.

*Stored information*
The process of comprehension is only complete when the words can be related to information which has been built up from past experience. The meaning of a new word has to be learnt.

## Expression of spoken language

*Selection of ideas*
A speaker has to decide first the general content of speech and then the means of expressing it. This will vary depending on the audience. For example, different words, intonation and syntax may be used when talking to a child rather than an adult.

*Selection of semantics (choice of words)*
The correct verbal label chosen to convey meaning may depend on where the speaker is and who the audience are. For example, one would choose different words to talk about women's lib at the Women's Institute than at the local pub.

*Selection of syntax (grammar)*
The order of the words chosen may again depend on the audience. The speaker may use correct grammar in some situations but in others may be less careful; for example, the difference between 'Who's that man talking to?' and 'To whom is that man talking?' may worry a purist, though in both sentences the meaning is plain.

*Motor patterns*
The ideas, words and grammar having been chosen, the appropriate sequence of motor patterns must be selected before articulation can take place, e.g. in the word 'car', the consonant 'c' precedes rather than follows the vowel.

*Articulation*
In association with breathing, the tongue, lips, palate and vocal cords must be correctly positioned and then moved for clear articulation.

## READING AND WRITING

Reading and writing follow a similar pattern. (See Fig. 4.2.)

**The basic structure of normal written language**

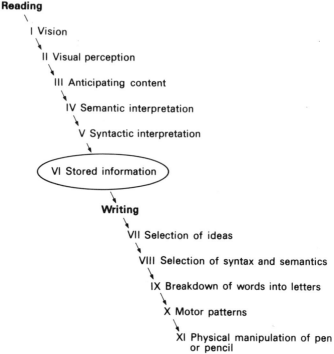

**Reading**

I Vision

II Visual perception

III Anticipating content

IV Semantic interpretation

V Syntactic interpretation

VI Stored information

**Writing**

VII Selection of ideas

VIII Selection of syntax and semantics

IX Breakdown of words into letters

X Motor patterns

XI Physical manipulation of pen or pencil

**Fig. 4.2**

## Reading

### Vision

In order to be able to read, visual acuity must be good enough to see the print. It is worth remembering the possibility of visual defect, and while this can usually be assumed to have been excluded, it should not be forgotten.

### Visual perception

The image on the retina must be translated by the brain into meaningful shapes and patterns, e.g. the individual components of a picture are distinguished from the background.

### Anticipating content

Many people who read quickly and many who do not read very well are helped by clues of punctuation, probability and context to identify words that they might otherwise misread, e.g. 'He threw a stick' is more likely than 'He threw a slick'.

*Semantic interpretation*
This relies either on recognising the pattern of the word because it has been seen so many times before, or on analysing it phonically. Words that are not spelt as they sound rely on the former or on the reader recognising that the pattern is similar to other words he may have seen.

*Syntactic interpretation*
The meaning of the sentence relies on the order of the words as in the syntactic interpretation of speech.

*Stored information*
A store of learned patterns is necessary in order for any of the preceding processes to be useful.

**Writing**

*Selection of ideas*
The writer must first decide what it is he is going to communicate.

*Selection of syntax and semantics*
The ideas then have to be translated into the words and sentence formation to be written. Sometimes this is the same structure used in speech but at other times the written word needs to be much more precise than the spoken word, e.g. when a solicitor is drawing up a document.

*Breakdown of words into letters*
Each word has to be broken down into the individual letters. Sometimes this is a well-learned pattern, at other times it has to be thought out by translating the phonetics to the written symbols.

*Motor patterns*
The brain must translate the language content of writing into its physical form. The correct motor patterns must therefore be selected.

*Physical manipulation of the pen or typewriter*
The process of writing is completed by putting pen to paper.

## ABNORMALITIES ARISING FROM HEAD INJURY

There are three main categories of speech and language disorder which may be caused by brain damage — dysphasia, dysarthria and dyspraxia.

*Dysphasia* is a disorder of language and may occur in comprehension, expression, reading or writing, although it usually affects all four. Thus a patient with receptive dysphasia may have a deficit in one or all of areas III, IV and V in Figure 4.1 and/or associated reading impairment in areas III, IV and V in Figure 4.2. A patient with expressive dysphasia will have a deficit in areas VII, VIII and IX in Figure 4.1 and/or a writing impairment in areas VII, VIII and IX in Figure 4.2.

*Dysarthria* is a physical disorder where the nerve supply to the musculature of articulation is inadequate. (See Fig. 4.1, 'Articulation'.) There are four possible types of dysarthria, three of which are commonly seen in a patient with head injury. These are upper motor neurone dysarthria, cerebellar dysarthria and extrapyramidal dysarthria. The dysarthria is seldom of one type alone in a patient with brain damage and is generally a mixture of all three.

*Dyspraxia* is a disorder of sequencing. Motor patterns of speech must be selected before words can be articulated. This includes the sequencing of articulatory movements, sounds within words, words within sentences and the logical formation of ideas. (See Fig. 4.1, Motor patterns.) Similarly the written word relies on the correct selection of motor patterns. (See Fig. 4.2, Motor patterns).

## ASSESSMENT OF DYSPHASIA

A brief description will be given of the levels of language ability that are considered mild, moderate or severe language disorders. The divisions are arbitrary and the range of patients seen by the therapist governs the way the disorders are graded. The patient need not be in the same category for comprehension, expression, reading and writing.

### Comprehension disorder

*Severe*
The patient is considered to have a severe comprehension difficulty if he fails some or all of the following tests:
(i) recognizing and selecting objects and pictures from sets of four or six
(ii) selecting these same objects and pictures by function
(iii) giving yes/no answers to simple questions and obeying simple commands

*Case example*
MH was only able to select two from a set of six objects, could not select at all by function, and was guessing at yes/no answers.

## Moderate
A moderate comprehension difficulty is said to exist when the patient fails:
  (i) to obey simple commands involving two elements or double commands, e.g. 'Put the kettle on and give me a biscuit'.
 (ii) in listening to a simple passage and giving yes/no answers
(iii) in answering questions where the apparently obvious answer is incorrect, e.g. 'Can everyone ride a bike?'
(iv) sorting out the key points in a passage read to him

*Case example*
WM could point out objects in a composite picture, but if asked to point to the door and window of the speech therapy department, he assumed that this command still referred to the picture. When answering yes/no questions he could only understand the nouns and the occasional verb and therefore was unable to respond correctly. However, he was able to answer yes or no to most of the questions from a short passage of text.

## Mild
The patient who fails only on the following is considered to have a mild comprehension difficulty:
  (i) obeying complex commands, some involving increased auditory retention, e.g. 'Show me the fat red-haired woman driving the small yellow car', and some involving comprehension of more sophisticated construction, e.g. 'If there is a red pencil, give me the tenpence piece'
 (ii) listening to a taped discussion and sorting out the two different viewpoints
(iii) understanding the inferences contained in a passage. At this level it is important to bear in mind the intellectual and educational ability of the patient before his accident

*Case example*
When being tested by the method above, RD picked up the tenpence piece even though there was no red pencil. Furthermore, he argued that although there was no red pencil there was a tenpence piece and therefore he must pick it up.

## Expression disorder

### Severe
The patient is considered to have a severe expressive difficulty if unable to:

   (i) imitate single words and phrases
  (ii) name objects and pictures or to give their function
 (iii) name items serially, e.g. days of the week, months of the year, or
 (iv) finish sentences, e.g. 'Pass the bread and ...'
  (v) give his name and address

*Case example*
When EH was asked to name a pencil she said 'I know — er — I know but I cannot say — er — you know — for paper.' However, she could complete sentences satisfactorily.

## Moderate

At this level the patient is expected to be able to attempt to:
  (i) give simple word definitions
 (ii) describe a picture using reasonable sentence structure
(iii) relate ideas and experience
(iv) retell a short passage

*Case example*
GC when describing a picture said, 'Oh yes, that one's a tree and that — that one there — is a [gesture] it's on top of the house, and there's a smoke.'

## Mild

If the patient is able to do all the exercises set for patients with moderate or severe disability, yet fails in some or all of the following, he is considered to have a mild expressive difficulty. He will be asked to:
  (i) describe people, places and activities
 (ii) give directions
(iii) give one-word answers to a quiz under pressure
(iv) give his own ideas in discussion.
  The subjects of these exercises must be kept within the patient's educational and intellectual ability.

*Case example*
AG, when asked to give a detailed description of a spirit level (a familiar tool of his trade), said, 'It has a bubble of water in it which tells you whether it's straight.' He was completely satisfied with this description.

## Reading disorder

*Severe*
The patient with a severe reading difficulty will fail on some or all of the following:

(i) recognising single letters
(ii) matching words to pictures
(iii) matching the spoken to the written word
(iv) giving yes/no answers to simple written questions

*Case example*
MD was able to match words to pictures but made semantic confusions in matching spoken to the written word, e.g. when asked to point to the word 'cat', she pointed to 'dog'.

*Moderate*
The patient with a moderate reading difficulty will succeed in the exercises set for severe reading difficulty, but fail on some or all of the following:
(i) reading simple stories and giving yes/no answers to questions
(ii) understanding written questions with more complicated syntax
(iii) reading a wide range of single words

*Case example*
WL was able to read a simple story and answer most of the questions correctly, but confused single words out of context, e.g. 'match' and 'watch'.

*Mild*
This is a difficult category to place patients in unless one knows their pre-morbid ability. They are assessed on their ability to:
(i) follow a written passage such as one might find in a newspaper
(ii) sort out the main ideas of such a passage
(iii) follow the line of argument in such a passage and do all this without taking undue time over it

*Case example*
CH was able to do all the items in this section but took three-quarters of an hour over an exercise which should have taken 10 minutes.

## Writing disorder

*Severe*
The patient is tested on his ability to:
(i) copy letters
(ii) write letters to dictation
(iii) write everyday words to dictation

*Case example*
NH spelt fish 'FISISH' and table 'FISABL'.

*Moderate*

The patient is required to:
  (i) write more unusual words to dictation
  (ii) put words into written sentences
  (iii) write a description of a picture or his job

*Case example*

JP was asked to write a description of his job in the RAF. 'I am in the RAF as a TAG. I AM A. TAG TAG is a tag. I am TAG since two yers.'

*Mild*

As for all assessments of mild impairment, a knowledge of the patient's standards before his accident is important. He will be asked to:
  (i) put complex words in sentences
  (ii) write word definitions
  (iii) spell polysyllabic words
  (iv) express idea and opinions in writing

There are several standardised assessments of dysphasia, such as the Minnesota Test for the Differential Diagnosis of Dysphasia and Porch Index of Communicative Ability (PICA).

## TREATMENT OF DYSPHASIA

All treatment as far as possible is based on developmental patterns. Babies hear sentences rather than single words, and their earliest attempts at communication are jargon that imitates intonation patterns of whole sentences. Therefore, a patient with a severe dysphasia is subjected to, and helped to produce, sentences from the start. Because these patients are having to relearn language with a damaged mechanism, it is necessary for them to learn within a rigid framework in the early days.

### Severe dysphasia

Much of the treatment in the early stages is based on very simple material such as a work card. This is a picture — any picture that provides interest — mounted on card with accompanying exercises in an envelope on the back. All the material is presented in simple sentences using a basic colour scheme: nouns and the definite and indefinite article in red, verbs and adverbs in green, adjectives in blue and all other words in black. The tense used is always the present continuous since this seems to be the natural choice when describing a picture. The exercises include a picture vocabulary of the main words appearing in the preceding exercises, and a written description of the picture which can be used for reading comprehension, reading aloud and as a basis for answering questions. There are three sets of questions relating to the passage. The first question requires yes/no answers, the second requires answers which reverse the question, e.g. 'Is the man running?' 'Yes, the man is running', and with the third question the patient is asked to select the appropriate written response from a choice. The picture can be used for an oral and written description, and also as the basis for discussion. The vocabulary can be learned and the words dictated to the patient, or he can be asked to put them into sentences. Having learned the basic vocabulary, the patient can be encouraged to work on his own with many of the exercises. With modifications the card can be used over and over again, reducing the amount of time spent by the therapist in 'preparation'.

The advantage of the work card system is that it uses the same vocabulary in many different ways, making the best use of repetition and overlearning. In each session the patient experiences continuous speech although with a limited vocabulary, rather than having an extensive vocabulary but not knowing how to use it. Most patients appreciate the more adult material even though the level is very simple, and they have a sense of achievement when a work card is finished.

## Moderate dysphasia

Treatment of a patient with moderate dysphasia should be much more flexible. At this stage the patient's own experiences will be included in the work. For example, a housewife would be using the sort of material relevant to her home life — family pictures, conversation about shopping, sequencing exercises involving household activities, etc. — while a garage mechanic will be working on material involving the vocabulary and language of his trade, naming tools used, describing how he would do jobs such as refitting an exhaust system or answering the telephone to customers.

The patient is encouraged to express his own ideas, to choose the material used and to build his vocabulary in the direction that he expects to find most useful. At this level communication is more important than precision, so that to be able to make someone understand is more important than the niceties of how that message is conveyed.

Speech therapy is no longer mainly confined to the speech therapy department, and the patient is encouraged to use his skills in a more open society. At first perhaps this will be by taking messages to other departments, but later he will go on shopping expeditions, visits to the library and if possible back to the place where he used to work.

**Mild dysphasia**

A patient with mild dysphasia has to be encouraged to compete with normal standards. The criterion of success is whether or not his level of understanding and communication would be accepted by people who do not know of his disability.

Most of the work is directed away from the obvious and concrete and involves discussion, argument and description of people, places and current events. Speed and accuracy are now considered important as is the ability to maintain the level of understanding and expression under pressure.

Discussions involving non-speech handicapped people are useful, so are quizzes with one word answers which have to be completed in a given time. Shopping expeditions at peak shopping hours, and buying a train ticket in the rush hour gives the patient practice in understanding and competing against the normal speed and level of conversation.

## HIGH LEVEL LANGUAGE DISORDER

Originally some of the patients were being readmitted to the Unit having failed at their old jobs. These patients were reassessed extensively and it was found that most of them fitted into the category that was labelled 'High Level Language Disorder'. This involved not just spoken and written language but a deficit in reasoning.

Conversationally these patients coped well, but their ability to follow instructions, argument and reasoning broke down under pressure, and their ability to produce reasoned argument and discusssion was poor. They were able to produce ideas, but if questioned were unable to defend or expand them. Their language, both oral and written, often seemed impressive at first, though inclined to be pedantic, but on closer examination there was considerable evidence of circumlocution, inappropriate use of words and phrases and dogmatic repetition. They were unable to complete satisfactorily exercises and games of logic and reasoning.

## ASSESSMENT

Assessment relies on a tape recorder and a flexible approach. The purpose of recording the assessment is that the therapist is not hampered by having to write down replies and does not have to ask the patient to repeat himself. The important parts are later transcribed, and analysed. The following assessment procedures are some of those devised for the age and intellectual range of the patients but may need to be varied for different situations.

1. A quiz with one-word answers to be completed in a given length of time

   It was found that many patients were unable to process terse questions and instructions if an immediate answer was required. For example, when asked the name given to a piece of land entirely surrounded by water, many gave the answer 'peninsular' or 'bay' although both these words are probably less commonly used than 'island'. When asked to list five fruits, it was not uncommon for the patient to give more than five or to repeat the first example twice, e.g. apple, pear, banana, orange, apple.

2. A problem situation was given which the patient read and then retold in order to ensure that he had understood the content

   He was asked what he would do in this situation. There is no right or wrong answer, and the therapist can accept his answer or question him until she is satisfied that his approach is reasonable and he has considered all the facts.

   The commonest errors here are that the patient has failed to draw inferences from the passage and therefore gives answers that are either impossible or inadequate.

3. Descriptions — The patient is asked to give concise descriptions of everyday objects

   He may know very well what a chair is, for example, but cannot convey the information to someone else. He may be able to conjure up a picture in his own mind, but lacks the ability to see the point of view of someone who has never seen one.

4. Sequences — Simple descriptive sequences such as making a cup of tea

   These often show how a patient is unable to marshall his thoughts and ideas clearly.

5. Expressing written ideas

   These can vary from describing his job, to giving his opinion about current events. His former educational ability must be taken into consideration as well as whether he has ever been accustomed to putting ideas into writing.

## TREATMENT

Treatment depends firstly on getting the patient to recognise that he has a problem. Tape recording is useful in the treatment of the patient who denies his previous statements if they are queried.

Unfortunately many patients are unable to recognise errors even if they are recorded and played back, and it is sometimes worth enlisting the help of someone of whom the patient has a high opinion — his boss, a close friend or the doctor — in order to help him to come to terms with his difficulty.

Working through each exercise, analysing what is wrong, encouraging insight and being prepared to agree in doubtful cases that the patient may be right, are all important, and perseverance, time and tact are all required.

Some of the exercises which we have found useful are listed below.

## Some treatment ideas

*Descriptions of pictures of people.* This brings in such things as imagining why a person might be in a particular mood and thoughts of what kind of work a person does, judging from their age, expression, clothes, etc. For example, a man with shoulder length hair and tie-dye t-shirt is unlikely to be a bank manager.

*Arguments.* The patient listens to recorded arguments. These should be fairly simple to start with, e.g. two people arguing about the way to the pub, with one taking a reasonable line of argument and the other one being unreasonable. This can be used for practice in disentangling two opposing opinions, in deciding why one is more logical than the other, in advancing the patient's own views on the argument and supplementing those ideas on the tape recorder, and also simple practice in following conversation at speed.

*First things first.* The patient is asked what is the first thing he would do in a given situation, e.g. if he were the only witness at the scene of a car crash. He has to justify why he would choose a particular course of action. In the example given, calling an ambulance, for instance, would be rather drastic action for a small bump. He has to learn to ask questions, to establish facts such as its being only a minor accident and to arrange his thoughts in order to be able to decide what is important and what is not.

*Discussing newspaper items.* This involves discussing what are the salient points, whether the article is biased and if so what might be the other side of the argument. In particular it is useful to explore those views and feelings with which the patient himself does not agree, to help him to be able to appreciate that differing points of view are not necessarily wrong.

*Exercises and games of reasoning.* There are many good educational games on the market which can be used with this group of patients. In particular those which involve categorising items where more than one property must be considered, linking apparently dissimilar items by a common factor, e.g. a pillar box and an apple are both red, and a tree and a baby are both living, and supplying the final element in a series, e.g. 1, 9, 17, 25 . . . where the number increases by a specific amount.

## ASSESSMENT OF DYSARTHRIA

Dysarthria is a physical disorder of speech caused by partial or complete damage to the nerves supplying the muscles involved in speech activity. This includes the supply to the lips, tongue, soft palate, mandible, cheeks, larynx and the respiratory mechanism. The disorder is seldom of one specific type following a head injury, so it is usually more useful to look at the individual aspects of speech rather than the symptoms of a particular dysarthric category. Assessment should include, therefore, consideration of breathing, phonation, articulation, resonance and intonation. On the whole, errors are consistent and a great deal of perseverance is needed on behalf of the patient to overcome the disorder.

### Breathing

Adequate breath control is essential for intelligible speech. The dysarthric patient may have difficulty inhaling sufficient air, taking short frequent breaths and only partially filling his lungs. It may be the exhalation that is affected where either the pressure of air is insufficient to vibrate the vocal cords, or a prolonged stream of air is not achieved, causing partial or total loss of volume. Treatment involves establishing adequate breathing patterns in isolation before speech is incorporated. The control of the diaphragm and intercostal muscles must be improved and strengthened, using techniques of resistance and practice in prolonging exhalation. It may be necessary to start this with the patient prone, progressing later to sitting and standing. Combining treatment with the physiotherapist is often of great assistance at this stage.

### Phonation

Partial paresis of the vocal cords is not uncommon after a head injury, especially if there has been prolonged intubation. This gives the voice a breathy quality and the patient may have difficulty increasing the volume. Treatment should include relaxation to reduce spasticity in the cords, by correct positioning of the head, manipulation, icing and relaxed breathing. Voicing should be gentle at first, gradually increasing the volume and using an open vowel such as 'ah'. Once adequate voice is established in isolation it should be included in speech, firstly in limited situations and later in more demanding ones until eventually the patient is able to cope in a crowded room or on the telephone.

## Articulation

This is frequently affected after a head injury although the disorder may only be mild depending on the amount of paralysis in the tongue and lips. Poor control of the tongue and lips may cause imprecise articulation of the individual sounds, inappropriate rhythm or excess speed. Where the individual sounds are inadequately articulated, treatment should begin with practice of the movements in isolation. If the patient is unable to make adequate closure of the lips, for instance, as for the sound b, this can be achieved by asking him to blow out his cheeks, or to hold a spatula between his lips, resisting attempts to remove it. Voicing can then be included and incorporated into simple words. This procedure should be repeated with all sounds, until polysyllabic words and continuous speech are mastered.

Inappropriate rhythm may be caused by an inability to vary the speed of articulation, as in scanning speech where all syllables are given equal emphasis, and articulation is slow and laboured. Treatment in this case involves increasing the ability to move the articulators at differing speeds. Excess speed of articulation often makes speech unintelligible, as the patient is unable to include all the sounds in the time available and the listener has difficulty processing what is said. The patient must be encouraged to slow down his speech and pronounce each syllable clearly, concentrating on the method rather than the content of speech.

## Resonance

The most common disorder of resonance in a head-injured patient is hypernasality caused by paresis of the soft palate. An inability to raise the soft palate prevents efficient execution of the majority of speech sounds, as the air escapes through the nasal rather than the oral aperture. Again, treatment should start with movements in isolation, facilitated by icing and resistance, and progress through individual sounds, simple and polysyllabic words to continuous speech.

## Intonation

Correct intonation patterns rely on adequate phonation and appropriate rhythm. They are affected in most cases of dysarthria and usually constitute the most difficult aspect to re-establish. Treatment is only effective if the patient understands what intonation is and can hear the difference between varying patterns. Using different patterns with the same words is often helpful in establishing intonation and shows how the mood of a sentence changes depending on the intonation employed, e.g. the difference between making a statement and asking a question.

## ASSESSMENT OF DYSPRAXIA

Dyspraxia is basically a disorder of sequencing. It may manifest itself in the articulation of a word, in the formation of a sentence or in the formulation of an idea. A patient with a dyspraxia will probably be unable to imitate, although errors will be likely to be inconsistent and he may sometimes succeed spontaneously where he had previously failed. Such patients often respond well to treatment.

The patient may be unable to perform any of the articulatory movements in isolation, despite adequate muscle power and intact nerve supply. Such a disorder would mean that the patient could chew and swallow, these movements being more automatic, but be unable to speak at all intelligibly.

The patient may be able to perform the movements in isolation but be unable to combine them into any form of speech. Thus he may put his lips together to form a 'b' sound but be unable to use his voice at the same time.

The patient may be able to combine all the movements required for articulation but be unable to use them in the correct order when speaking. Thus a patient might say B C B instead of B B C, knowing it to be incorrect but being unable to remedy it.

The patient may be able to say individual words but be unable to put them together in the correct order. This may drastically alter the meaning of the sentence or even render it unintelligible.

The patient may be unable to put his thoughts into words, although not because of a language deficiency. Thus he may say 'Yes' when he means 'No', or 'It's raining' when he means 'It's fine'. Such a patient may frequently converse adequately and then when questioned may apparently refuse to answer. He therefore gives the impression of failing to cooperate, particularly as he is probably unable to alter the inappropriate response.

The patient may be unable to sort out his ideas correctly and so cannot verbalise them. Such a patient, although being able to perform an activity such as making a cup of tea, will be unable to describe the same activity in the correct order, for example, he may say, 'Put the kettle on. Put the tea in the pot. Pour the tea into the cup. Put the boiling water in the pot.' This often means that the patient himself becomes confused and is therefore largely unable to follow through any train of thought.    Other associated dyspraxias are occasionally seen, such as an inability to use facial expression at will, an inability to use gesture and, more commonly, an inability to manipulate a pen when writing.

Dyspraxia is rarely seen in isolation in head-injured patients and is therefore difficult to diagnose. It is often impossible to assess how much a patient's speech is affected by either a dyspraxia or dysarthria, in a case where both are present. The assessment follows the same form as a dysarthria assessment initially, asking the patient to perform individual articulatory movements, and to repeat monosyllabic and polysyllabic words. If there are no signs of physical weakness, or if any weakness there may be is insufficient to warrant the disability, or if the patient is able to perform adequately at times but fails at other times, then it may be suspected that the disability is of a dyspraxic rather than dysarthric origin. Similarly, if the patient is able to perform quite well in the language assessment but makes inconsistent errors, which he may well recognise, such as putting words in the wrong order or being unable to sort out his thoughts correctly, then the possibility of a dyspraxia must be considered.

## TREATMENT OF DYSPRAXIA

The basis of the treatment of dyspraxia lies in relearning actions which should come naturally with or without conscious thought, but which are no longer under voluntary control. Constant repetition is therefore essential, building up performance from residual abilities. The individual articulatory movements can be facilitated by working from involuntary movements, e.g. opening the mouth can be stimulated from a yawn, pursing the lips from blowing or whistling, tongue movements from licking the lips, soft palate movements from puffing out the cheeks etc. Proprioceptive neuromuscular facilitation (PNF) techniques can also be useful for stimulating individual articulators. It may sometimes be necessary to remove the communication element of speech, when the patient is unable to perform the individual sounds. This can be achieved by encouraging the patient to sigh aloud for instance or laugh or cough, gradually introducing related sounds more nearly associated with normal speech, e.g. starting with a cough the 'k' sound can be introduced until eventually the word car is achieved. At this stage of treatment it is important that all modalities are used to reinforce the motor activity and bring it under voluntary control. The movements required to produce sounds should be explained, pictures and diagrams drawn, movements imitated using a mirror and tactile stimulation given to the articulators. Gradually the sounds should be incorporated into words and comparisons made between similar words, e.g. the difference between bed and bad, cat and act, irrelevant and irreverent. If the patient has difficulty in putting the words in the correct order or assembling his ideas, activities in sequencing non-verbal material should be practised, such as sorting out a story in pictures, or providing the missing element of a pictorial series, or matching individual components to the correct composite picture.

This will lead on to verbal exercises, such as putting the words of a muddled sentence into the correct order, expressing the ideas of a long sentence in a few concise words as in a telegram, or sorting out two stories that have been muddled together.

The treatment of writing dyspraxia follows a similar line, facilitating precise control of the pen by practising basic writing patterns, incorporating them in letters and finally words.

## MEMORY DISORDERS

Memory traces appear to be laid down all over the brain and disorders of memory after a severe head injury are therefore common. They vary from mild problems such as a difficulty in remembering the occasional instruction to a prolonged or even permanent post-traumatic amnesia. Any memory disorder is likely to affect the patient's response to treatment in all departments and it is therefore essential that a reliable memory is established as soon as possible. Since memory and language disorders are often closely associated — the patient who has not fully understood an instruction will have great difficulty in committing it to memory adequately — the treatment of such disorders is often undertaken by the speech therapists at RAF Chessington.

Although there are standardised assessments of memory in several psychological tests, we decided to devise our own assessment so that it could be as functional to our needs as possible. Memory performance varies with age and the test was therefore standardised over only a small percentage of the population but one which correlated closely to the majority of our patients. The material used is particularly relevant to their life-style and interests. When assessing patients we are looking broadly at three main factors: memory of events which occurred both before and after the brain injury; performance in both the short term — up to five minutes after the initial stimulus — and in the long term — 24 hours after the initial stimulus; memory of material when the patient is firstly unaware and secondly aware that he will have to recall it.

Since many of the patients are suffering additional problems from the head injury, e.g. visual impairment or language deficit, memory is assessed in all modalities. For example, several items are tested in auditory, verbal and visual modalities. It is often impossible to diagnose accurately the nature and extent of a memory impairment but it is usually possible to indicate the severity of the disorder and how it is likely to affect general performance.

Treatment obviously varies according to the handicap but an additional important influence is the patient's pre-morbid memory techniques. The patient himself is probably unaware of the methods he used and treatment is therefore largely a case of trying out different techniques until a suitable one is found for each individual.

The patient with a mild memory disorder will usually require no treatment, as he will either learn to overcome any difficulties himself or they will recover spontaneously. Such a patient will probably have trouble in remembering things from day to day, although his memory may be reliable for some hours. If prompted, he is likely to remember what he is unable to recall spontaneously. Such treatment as may be necessary will probably involve no more than helping the patient become aware of the problem and encouraging him to discover ways of helping himself. Usually the most effective way of overcoming this sort of disorder is for the patient to write down everything he wishes to remember and then refer to his notebook frequently, for instance every hour on hearing the clock strike. It may also help if the therapist talks to his family to explain the difficulties he is likely to experience.

The patient with a moderate disorder will normally have great difficulty in remembering events from day to day. Many memories will also fade after a couple of hours or even within an hour, and his ability to learn from experience will be limited. Thus all treatment, in whatever department, will be adversely affected and each activity will have to be constantly repeated before any useful learning occurs. Many of these patients appear to have difficulty absorbing material initially, so treatment is based largely on stimulating input rather than facilitating output. Thus in many cases comprehension exercises are relevant, e.g. the patient is read or reads a passage, picks out the most important facts, writes them down and uses this list to remind him of the content of the passage. This can later be internalised so that he no longer needs to rely on the written prompts and can use the technique when listening to a conversation or taking instructions. Many patients find this exercise very difficult and need a great deal of practice in merely deciding on the most important points, before they can attempt to commit them to memory. Another technique which is sometimes successful is associating items with stimuli which are more relevant to the individual, such as colours or musical instruments. When trying to store information the patient pictures the item in a particular colour or linked to a particular musical instrument and then on recalling the colour or instrument, the memory of the information will be stimulated. Clearly this requires a certain amount of ingenuity and application on the part of the patient. Having discovered a technique which helps, the patient must practise it constantly, so that eventually he is not really aware that he is using it. This means that the therapist must think of a wide variety of activities such as flash cards with pictures of a few items, Kim's game, written passages, composite pictures, taking map directions, etc.

The patient with a severe memory disorder will be disorientated in time and place, will probably have an incomplete memory of his past life and a memory span of not more than an hour and usually much less. Such patients are very confused and often completely unaware that they have a problem.

*Case example*
The following is a copy of a letter sent by a patient with a severe memory disorder but minimal associated handicaps.
'Dear Mum,
How are you, I am well. I will come home as soon as possible. Your ever loving son John Peter Smith. I hope I will see you as soon as possible. Your ever loving son. I am at RAF Chessington but I will be home as soon as possible. Your ever loving son John Peter Smith.' On re-reading this letter the patient was completely satisfied and unaware that he had repeated himself several times since his memory span was only a few seconds.

Clearly such a disorder precludes any formal conventional therapy until the patient is able to remember even for long enough to complete a simple task. With a severe memory disorder the patient approaches an activity as if for the first time on each repetition. He must, therefore, be very confused and probably frightened, as he has no experience to which to refer. If he has any awareness of the problem he will lack confidence in his ability, which he may counter with excessive aggression which exacerbates the difficulties. It is essential, therefore, that he builds up a relationship with one person in a stable environment, so that he gains confidence in extremely limited surroundings and can begin to tackle the enormous problems. As far as possible treatment of such patients is confined to the ward and one department, so he meets one or two therapists only. These patients are encouraged to learn the names of the therapists so that they recognise them as individuals and so that later the same names used elsewhere will have some meaning. Gradually the environment is widened and new people introduced, ensuring all the time that the patient maintains confidence in his surroundings. Whenever he is taken from one place to another his attention is drawn to the route and the distinguishing features of the buildings, so that he will eventually be able to take himself around, establishing the beginnings of independence. It is often necessary to use techniques such as visual association to remember the names of the people. Thus the name Churchill would be depicted as a church on a hill, Karr as a car and Palmer as palm trees or the palm of a hand. The associations can be very obvious or obscure, so long as the patient finds them useful. For those patients who are unable to use associations constant repetition and simple rote learning may be the only alternative. This is inclined to become monotonous, however, more for the therapist or relative rather than the patient as he will not realise he has done the same thing over and over again.

An association technique used to great advantage with one patient was linking the activity with numbers and rhyming pictures. The patient had been extremely disorientated and was unable to complete even a simple well-rehearsed activity successfully. Thus when cleaning her teeth in the morning she might forget to use the toothpaste. When given a structured framework she was able to cope. Starting with the number 1 she chose a word which rhymed, e.g. sun. A picture of a sun was drawn and inside this a picture of a toothbrush. The number 2 was associated with 'shoe', pictured with toothpaste

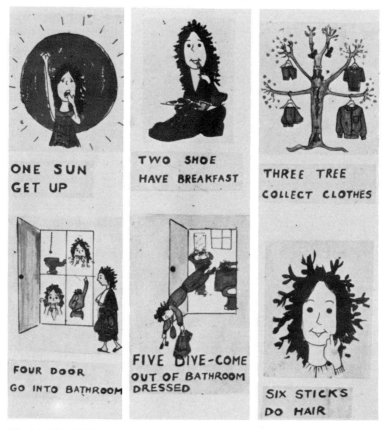

**ONE SUN GET UP**

**TWO SHOE HAVE BREAKFAST**

**THREE TREE COLLECT CLOTHES**

**FOUR DOOR GO INTO BATHROOM**

**FIVE DIVE-COME OUT OF BATHROOM DRESSED**

**SIX STICKS DO HAIR**

**Fig. 4.3** Visual aid produced to help patient complete her toilet successfully.

coming out of it. Number 3 was associated with a tree whose branches were producing water, and so on, until the process of cleaning teeth was completed. This system, although very successful with this patient, was no help to several others with similar problems, emphasising the fact that each patient, with the therapist's help, must devise his own system (Fig. 4.3).

## GENERAL MANAGEMENT

When a patient is referred for treatment, one of the major considerations is thorough assessment. However, unless the therapist is adept at presenting test material in an informal and easy way, this is not necessarily the first thing to do. It is often more important to build up a good relationship first, giving the patient an opportunity to get used to the place and the people with whom he or she will be working. On the other hand, there are patients who like to feel that formal speech therapy has been started and these people may be encouraged by having a structured assessment at the first session.

Whenever assessment is attempted, it is important to appreciate that there may be associated disabilities which will affect the patient's speech and language. These are either physical problems resulting from the head injury or alterations in mood and motivation.

Physical problems which may affect communication are those concerned with sight, hearing, head control, and oral movements.

### Visual defects

These can range from total blindness to slight visual imperception. Total blindness requires some ingenuity in preparing treatment material that does not rely on vision, but at least the problem is easily identifiable. Some visual field defects, however, e.g. tunnel vision and homonymous hemianopia, are not so easily apparent and it may be necessary for the patient to have a perimetry test for accurate diagnosis. In such cases, material should only be presented within the patient's visual field. Visual imperception is common in patients suffering from brain damage. This may manifest itself in an inability either to switch from one line to the next in reading or to recognise a slightly ambiguous picture or to copy a diagram correctly or simply to manoeuvre round a room adequately. For example, the patient may sit down before reaching a chair or try to step high over a crack in the floor. If there is a suspected defect of visual perception the patient should either be referred elsewhere for detailed assessment or the speech therapist herself may be able to diagnose the type and extent of the difficulty using the standard tests available. In the treatment of these patients visual material should be used with caution.

**Hearing defects**

Simple audiometric screening can pick up obvious defects of hearing, although an Ear, Nose and Throat Department will produce a more detailed audiogram. The possibility of hearing loss often seems to have been overlooked and can add greatly to a patient's difficulties. There may, however, be no actual hearing loss but a difficulty in perceiving sound, e.g. the patient hears the sound at the correct intensity but cannot make sense of it. An example of this is a patient who listened to a tape recording of everyday noises, e.g. a car starting, a bird singing, a tap running, and identified each one as a musical instrument. Quite often this difficulty is simply a manifestation of the patient's general confusion, and improves with the patient's increasing confidence in his surroundings. Whatever the cause, it is important to identify the problem in order, firstly to tackle it and secondly to ensure that all material is backed up initially by increased use of other modalities, e.g. sight and touch.

**Head control**

Poor head control, particularly when associated as it usually is with other severe physical problems, can interfere with the patient's communication. He may not be able to watch the speaker's face and so will miss many clues of facial expression and gesture. If the larynx is not in the mid-line position there is undue strain on the vocal cords which may cause voice problems and finally the head may be slumped forward so that speech becomes less intelligible and articulation of some consonants, particularly palatal plosives, can be affected.

**Oral movements**

There may be specific oral injury affecting speech, such as a broken jaw, missing teeth or dentures and occasionally severe mutilation of the tongue.

**Mood and motivation**

Most of the alterations in mood and motivation are a result of widespread rather than focal damage causing such problems as euphoria, depression, inflated ego, aggression, diminished responsibility, intolerance and poor insight. Many of these are exacerbated by a long stay in hospital or by overprotection at home.

No matter how hard the therapist works, unless the patient is well motivated towards recovery there is unlikely to be any significant progress. Many of the problems associated with a head injury affect motivation. For example, patients may be euphoric or depressed or have swings between the two moods. A euphoric patient who has an unrealistic feeling of well-being may admit his problems but be unable to regard them seriously. He may believe that he will soon be better, that his job is being 'held open' for him or that he will have adequate compensation and need never work again. A depressed patient may be unable to lift himself above a gloomy contemplation of his state in order to work at improving it.

A patient with poor insight into his problems may not recognise his limitations. He may want to discontinue treatment because he thinks he has no further need of it or he may want to concentrate on one small, possibly unimportant area to the exclusion of all else. He will be unable to monitor his own progress and therefore will need constant supervision. Later he will be unable to appreciate possible difficulties in finding employment and in social relationships.

Many patients who have been in intensive care for some time or at home surrounded by loving, worrying relatives, may have an inflated ego. They may want the whole of the therapist's attention and will not mix well in a group for treatment. They may be aggressive towards other patients and intolerant of mistakes while accepting or not recognising their own errors.

External factors that should be taken into consideration when treating patients are such things as the weather, the drugs they are on and their personal relationships.

**Functional prognosis**

Realistic prognosis relies heavily on the kind of factors, physical and emotional, mentioned above.

In addition to handicaps resulting from a head injury, various pre-morbid factors must be taken into account. For instance, the original intelligence of the patient will affect his progress. However, a greater intelligence does not necessarily correspond with a higher level of achievement. The expectations of an intelligent patient may be too high and he may be dissatisfied with a lower level of achievement. On the other hand, he will probably have a greater potential to realise and may therefore make more progress in the end.

Pre-morbid personality is also an influential factor. A placid person may find it easier to accept his problems but may also lack the necessary application to improve, while an ambitious person may find it hard to accept the handicap but retain high motivation.

# 5

# Educational therapy

## INTRODUCTION

At Chessington a unique and unusual post of educational therapist was first established full time in 1973. The prime task of the therapist was to assist in the assessment and treatment of those patients with severe intellectual deficit. The assessments were to be conducted on conventional educational lines as far as the disability would allow, but once the problem of either retrieval of old memories or inability to acquire new information had been identified, then both conventional and unconventional teaching patterns were used to overcome this handicap. In common with the social worker and the other non-medical members of the rehabilitation team the educational therapist brought with her the jargon of her own profession, and one of the prime problems for members of the rehabilitation team was in understanding the jargon of the others. To help this, the team approach, regular weekly meetings and an informal atmosphere in the unit among the therapy staff proved invaluable, but even so it took some months and even years before the value of the role was fully realised.

It was also appreciated very early on through the course of the Chessington study, that an enormous amount of existing information could be obtained about the patient's previous background by going back through service records, for uniquely in the three services all recruits are subjected to a battery of tests on selection and by a suitable approach these results can be obtained. Previous work (Vivash 1972) had established that the standard conventional medical tests correlated extremely well with standard medically used tests. So for the service population who had suffered brain damage the unit was in the unique position of having accurate assessment of the pre-morbid intellectual ability and, in many cases, also pre-morbid performance of the patients who subsequently came to it. Much of the experience gained in the educational therapy department served as a model for showing methods of integration of new approaches into what had hitherto been a relatively rigid structure confined effectively to medical and paramedical members only.

The therapist who was appointed realised very early that the medical jargon was quite a barrier and so also was the jargon that she used. 'But, armed with a medical dictionary and aided by the tolerant explanation of doctors, nurses, speech therapists and anyone within questioning distance, my vocabulary increased by leaps and bounds. I learned to cope with such tongue-satisfying words as perseveration, echolalia and negativism. I even began to have a dim understanding of psychologists' reports — 'His errors are due to a visual agnosia linked with a parieto-occipital dysfunction.'

The therapist found that certain aspects of practical nursing problems had to be learnt rapidly, and both she and the rest of the team in the department regularly practised the art of resuscitation and first aid. They learned to cope with epileptic fits, to manipulate wheelchairs and how to remove food from the mouth of a choking patient. It is difficult to overemphasise the points that have thus far been enumerated, because they apply not only to an inexperienced educational therapist coming into the field of medical rehabilitation, but with equal force to other members of the rehabilitation team who may not have had any form of training even in first aid or resuscitation; a certain basic knowledge of all these skills should be common throughout the team. These points also serve to underline the enormous problems that relatives who are equally naive as far as medical training is concerned have to face when for the first time they take home relatives who have been handicapped. It is only too easy to assume, from the lofty attitudes of familiarity, that everybody else has the same fluency with medical jargon and routine.

Two further points came up as part of the therapist's basic reactions to this new situation. She learned how to react normally to patients who at the time that she met them, from her point of view, were decidedly abnormal: she found that it was important not to talk down to, ignore or talk across a patient with communication difficulties. She became aware of the usefulness of visual cues such as facial expression and hand movements in helping comprehension, and also that the trick of rephrasing any statement in as many ways as possible was an invaluable aid to communication. This last skill came more easily to the educational therapist since it was a simplified form of a basic teaching approach, so here the information was reversed and for many members of the team there was the deepening appreciation of the fact that there were many methods of communication with brain-damaged patients which hitherto had not been explored.

## ASSESSMENT

All members of the Forces sit a battery of tests at their respective recruit selection centres before they enter service. In the cases of Service patients these records provide an invaluable standard which, once retrieved, become available for inclusion in the assessments. Although the scope and number of subtests covered by the three services vary, some elements are common to all of them: (1) a non-verbal IQ score; (2) vocabulary/English score; (3) an arithmetic grading; (4) an overall ability grading. Correlations between these various tests of the services have been calculated in an interservice test project conducted by the psychological research departments concerned. An equivalent notional overall IQ score could therefore be calculated from the overall ability grading of any individual. The original test results and those achieved subsequently were graded on five-point scales, though in most cases the actual quotient was recorded as well. Commercially available and established tests were chosen for the education assessments. These were Raven's progressive matrices (which allow for slight deterioration in performance with age), the Mill Hill vocabulary scales (which allow for improvement up to the age of 65), Vernon's graded mathematics test (which has a wide application to resettlement assessment) and the Cattell IQ which eventually became more useful for discovering high-level verbal reasoning difficulties. Where appropriate, tests such as the National Foundation for Educational Reading Research tests and the Porteus maze tests were also included. All these educational assessments were graded on a five-point scale and it was shown (Vivash 1973) that the degree of accuracy was well within the scope of the proven correlations between the commercial tests and the main subtests of the three services. It was recognised that many of the servicemen would normally have received education aimed at improving many of these basic abilities and this was one of many reasons for treating information gained with extreme caution.

Another problem with the initial assessment was the decision as to the timing of the tests. Newly arrived patients were frequently confused, disorientated and still in a post-traumatic amnesic state and might perform very badly in a test with which they could cope much better in a subsequent week. However, some form of compromise was essential since the longer the wait the longer treatment was postponed and the more pointless the testing became. It was also felt important to start building a rapport with the patients as soon as possible. Many patients (particularly the 'brighter' ones) viewed the IQ tests with great suspicion, since they recognised them from their own past experience within the service. Eventually a compromise was reached and testing was done during the second week, using the first week as an introduction to the department and staff. Wherever possible, test material was read to those with poor sight, though it was appreciated that this could cause testing unreliability and invalidity.

Testing also caused problems in space and time. For continuity and reliability and cross-correlation it was important to use the same tester. It was necessary to have a quiet room with space for both the tester and several patients at once to sit and write comfortably. The whole range of tests could take between three to 12 hours to complete. The only test with a time limit was Cattell's IQ. Eventually the education clerk, who had been trained to administer the tests, fitted four desks in the library and conditions, though not ideal, were adequate (see Fig. 5.1).

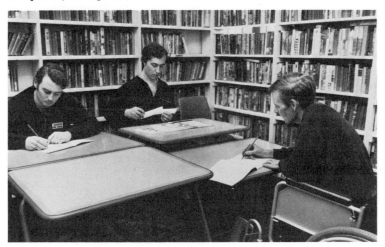

**Fig. 5.1**   Testing conditions in the education library.

*Other pre-injury information*
The recruit selection records also include valuable pre-morbid information about a person's family, social background, physical appearance hobbies and interests. There is also information about the educational achievements, school and job records, and scores in a variety of aptitude tests. Information about subsequent education, training and even character can also be obtained up to the time of injury. From this, it was possible to set a realistic level for retraining; though some patients were found able to exceed their previous standards (perhaps as a result of the very intensive interest and one-to-one coaching). New areas of interest or ability were sometimes discovered which could compensate for lost ones or lead to useful

resettlement. Special areas of difficulty such as arithmetic could be identified and if necessary worked upon. Pre-morbid material available for non-service patients was obtained from past schools, educational achievement, and family and employers' comments, but though more limited and subjective, it was still of value in attempting to set realistic goals.

All assessments were recorded and any relevant comments about the patient's approach to the tests, ability to concentrate and general willingness to cooperate, were added. Where known, the actual numerical quotient was also recorded. Recruit selection scores were also recorded in graph form to obtain an immediate visual comparison. The patient was retested at intervals of about three months so the new levels of achievement could be noted. Improvement varied from patient to patient, and it was very rare for a patient to show none. Whether the improvement could be attributed to the work done in the section or not, rapid improvement was more typical in non-verbal than verbal areas. Figure 5.2 shows the graph of the educational assessments of a male patient, aged 17, who fell, sustained a head injury and was unconscious for two weeks with a PTA of about eight to ten weeks.

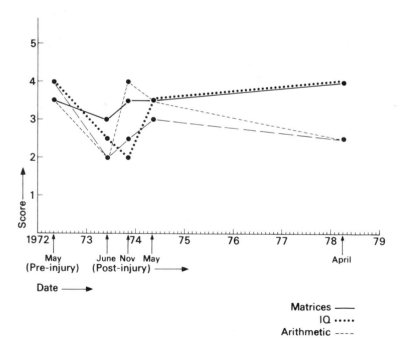

Fig. 5.2 Education assessment of head-injured patients.

# TREATMENT

## The education centre

The Education Centre consisted of a fully equipped classroom, library, large semi-partitioned general studies/coffee room, small sound-proof booth, three offices, small kitchen and two toilets. Figure 5.3 shows.another part of the education library. Most of the equipment needs for items costing up to £150 (other than those supplied through service sources) could be purchased. More expensive items were given, begged, borrowed or 'self-purchased'.

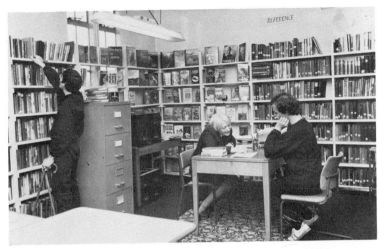

**Fig. 5.3**   The education library. (The educational therapist is in the middle!)

## Physical disabilities

The majority of the head-injury patients had some form of physical disability which involved simple, but necessary, practical considerations. Since independence was encouraged, exercise books, writing equipment, programmed learning machines and other self-study material were stored, whenever possible, within easy reach of the wheelchair patient. Desks and tables were high enough for a wheelchair to fit under and spaced out so that wheelchairs could pass by. Writing implements were available in assorted diameters for disabled hands to grasp. Sometimes a patient had to relearn the motor skills of writing almost from nothing, or learn to write with his non-dominant hand. The series of commercial exercises published by ESA for training in motor skills were of some help (see Fig. 5.4). The process was often slow and devoured sheets of paper. The equipment included an electric typewriter with a keyboard adaptor to prevent fingers slipping, for those for whom writing was impractical.

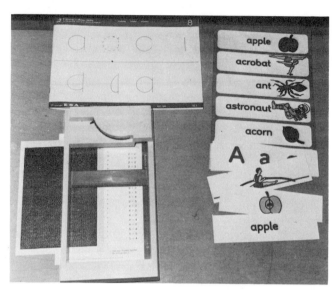

**Fig. 5.4** Relearning old basic skills. Top left — ESA training in motor skills. Bottom left — SRA arithmetic fact kit.

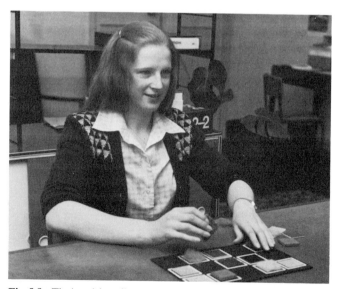

**Fig. 5.5** The 'touch board'.

The most difficult patients in this category had extensive visual/or perceptual problems. Despite the use of a talking book and tape recorder, treatment was usually verbal and one-to-one and made extensive demands on the time of both staff and patients. Figure 5.5 shows a 'touch board' which was covered with squares of materials ranging in feel from smooth glass to soft fur and rough matting. The idea could easily be developed to provide not only memory and perception tests for the blind, but also stimulate imaginative conversation. Large-print books were available in the library, and some of the material, including the tests, was rewritten in letters four inches high.

The incumbent of the post was new and had some pertinent comments to make.

*Language problems*
I remember too well my first encounter with a dysphasic patient, the essence of which is reproduced below, as a lesson in how not to do it.
'Good morning. Are you the new patient?'
'Yes.'
'You must be Michael, then?'
'Yes.'
'Sit down, Michael. I'm going to say some words to you and I'd like you to explain their meaning to me. Do you understand?'
'Yes.'
'Before we start, Michael, when did you arrive?'
'Yes.'
I kept a straight face and ploughed on.
'Could you tell me what an apple is, Michael? . . . What does an apple look like?'
'It's red.'
'Good, good, well done. What do you do with an apple? What do you use it for?'
'You drive it . . . that is to say, if you're driving, when you get there, you use it, if you see what I mean.'
I didn't see at all. In desperation I gave him a sheet of paper and asked him to write down the meanings of the words given. The essence of his reply is as follows:

| Word given | Michael's answer |
| --- | --- |
| Hat | Tea |
| Sad | Walk |
| Upset | Think |
| Fight | Walk |
| See | Think |
| Carry on | Thinking |
| Frighten | Water |

| | |
|---|---|
| Scent | Walk |
| Disease | Thinker |
| Mix | Midderl |
| Boast | Spoon |
| Trick | Thinker |

Michael had severe language difficulties in both expression and comprehension. In the early stages of treatment, patients with severe language problems spent a large part of their day in the Speech Therapy department although we would sometimes in Education provide back up work in reading and writing, increasingly in the later stages. It was often a problem to find suitable work which was not childish in format. The Science Research Associates (SRA) study programmes such as 'Reading for Understanding' and 'Research Laboratory' and 'Spelling Word Power Laboratory' were found to be invaluable, particularly for testing skills at different levels. The Clifton audio visual reading programme (see Fig. 5.6), which is phonetically based, enabled patients to work at their own pace. Provided the patient was sufficiently aware to be able to operate a tape recorder, this could be done alone in a sound-proof booth.

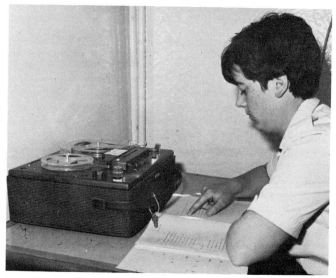

**Fig. 5.6**   The Clifton audio-visual reading programme.

## Programmed learning

Over the years much programmed learning material was acquired, both linear and branched examples. Not only were they time-savers for the instructor, but their pre-structured nature ensured a disciplined approach (though limited to the skill and aim of the programmer). Many head-injured patients seemed to respond well to the highly structured programmes, and the repetitive nature of the linear programme was particularly useful where a patient had some form of memory impairment. The Bingley Tutor and Royal Navy NAMET programmes in English and arithmetic, for example, provided basic repetitive one-word answer work. The Autotutor branched programmes on the following of instructions and on reading and comprehension provided more advanced and less repetitive work. Where some patients were physically unable to write it was particularly advantageous that the machines with their choice of answers could be worked by the pressing of buttons. One shy patient in particular loved this form of programmed learning. The machine did not frighten him as people did. Figure 5.7 shows a patient at work on a high level programme in the Autotutor Mark II.

**Arithmetic**
Work with discalculic patients ranged from the use of playing cards to reinforce numeracy to much higher level work on decimals and fractions. This was aided by the Army EPC programmes and the Royal Navy NAMET programmes and the recently produced RAF Calculations books. Counters were used effectively with the highly repetitive SRA Arithmetic Fact Kit (Fig. 5.4). A simple machine provided with this kit forced the user to work at a certain set pace. As the user felt more confident in, for example, adding a list of numbers

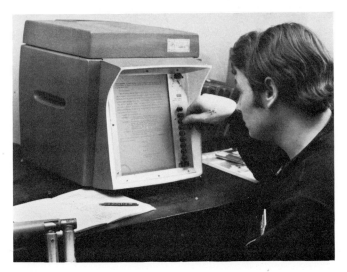

**Fig. 5.7**   The Autotutor Mark II.

ranging from 2 add 0, to 5 add 4, he could increase the machine's speed, until eventually he was working at his own maximal pace. However, the concentration required was considerable and it was countereffective to let a patient work on the machine for more than 10 minutes at a time.

One basic priority was to enable a patient to have sufficient arithmetic to cope with everyday life. Rote repetitive learning such as the recitation of multiplication tables or work on the Fact Kit seemed to produce more effective and faster results with the severely brain-damaged than attempting to explain the concepts and reasoning behind arithmetic. It seemed to be of critical importance that a patient should always arrange his work in the same rigid organised manner than that he understood why he was doing it that way. Similarly the application of that arithmetic whether it was reading a train timetable, budgeting or adding the price of goods in a shop seemed to require the same rigid and repetitive approach. Patients did not seem to become as bored with work of this nature as expected, despite the fact that the patients working at these simplest levels often also had concentration difficulties.

The SRA Computapes provide cassette learning packages with accompanying test and exercise books. Although aimed at a lower age group, the Computapes were nevertheless sufficiently lively and of the right length and difficulty, to keep most patients stimulated and interested. Figure 5.8 shows the Computapes in use. This programme, like many of the others, saved some of the time spent on repetitive one-

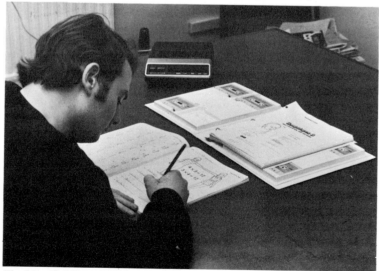

Fig. 5.8   SRA Computapes.

to-one work which would otherwise have been necessary. Finally, it was important to remember to use any remaining number bonds or skills a patient might have — one patient who was struggling to work out 2 × 19 on paper, answered immediately and correctly when asked for 'double top, triple nineteen and bull!'

### Previous trades
Sometimes a patient needed to revise the background knowledge of his previous job. (The practical skill would be assessed as far as possible in the occupational therapy department.) Here the need for the education therapist to be a jack-of-all trades was at its most marked since the jobs to be assessed ranged from a naval stoker to a lawyer. Testing the academic knowledge and memory of an ex-anaesthetist was virtually impossible; nevertheless, comment on his powers of concentration was relevant. Finally, where a patient was obviously unable to return to his last job, it was sometimes worth investigation whether he could still do the job before the last one, perhaps before he joined the service.

### Reasoning
It was sometimes considered important to stimulate a patient mentally in other fields and where possible practice was provided in non-verbal thinking, possibly with the use of logic games such as Mastermind, logic blocks, jigsaw puzzles, mazes or even advanced noughts and crosses (in three dimensions). Learning Development Association provided useful material for work on concept development. Even if non-verbal games achieved little else, they sometimes provided status to a patient with difficulties in expression by showing staff as well as fellow patients that he could still reason well even if he could not easily communicate that reasoning.

### Group work
Patients with higher grade speech or comprehension loss, or those who had progressed well, were often grouped together in the later stages to encourage verbalisation, problem-solving or self-confidence. They joined in play-reading, quizzes and discussion groups, sometimes helped by the use of record players, tape recorders, loop projectors, slides with tape commentaries or films (which were usually supplied free by advertisers). Figure 5.9 shows a patient controlling the loop projector. Group work provided the most exhausting, satisfying, but sometimes frustrating sessions in the timetable. The interaction between patients, both helpful and obstructive, provided valuable insight into the way in which they were probably going to survive or

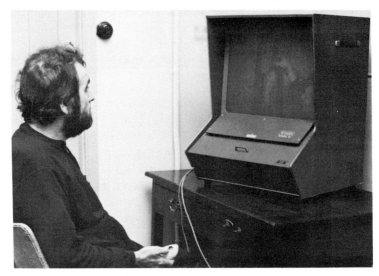

**Fig. 5.9** The loop projection.

otherwise in their future social and working life (whether sheltered or not) outside the unit.

Group work usually took place in the General Studies Room. This was also a communal coffee room where patients, including non-head-injured patients, gathered at coffee breaks to read newspapers as well as drink coffee. Figure 5.10 shows the Medical Social Worker (whose office was adjacent to the room) chatting to one of the patients during

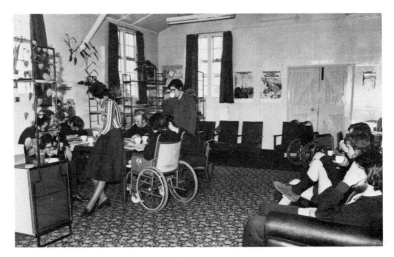

**Fig. 5.10** General studies room — coffee break.

such a break. Non-head-injury patients were occasionally encouraged to join in the group sessions and sometimes provided useful contrast and differing viewpoints.

Play-reading was particularly popular, especially if the plays were funny, short, and within the patient's comprehension. Once the ice had been broken (usually by a carefully chosen extrovert patient) even the patient who had difficulty in reading seemed not only unselfconscious but sometimes eager to take part. It was pleasantly surprising to find how tolerant the others could be of the slow, hesitant or monotonous reader (though plays with long speeches were avoided whenever possible). As a group progressed, its members were encouraged to comment on the quality of plays and characters and discuss how they would react in a similar situation.

### Learning new skills

Learning new skills could sometimes help to compensate for lost ones (such as trying to replace writing or even speech). Frequently, because of reduced job prospects, training a patient in a new skill would be started by bringing him up to the academic level needed for retraining or by investigating alternative aptitudes, interests or abilities. For example, there were often patients who needed training to bring them up to the standard required to pass the arithmetic tests for the Government Skills Centre courses. It was sometimes necessary to do rapid and intensive research into the academic skills required of a variety of trades. Occasionally it was possible to have a patient working on clerical or library duties in the department itself. Again commercial programmes helped to widen what was available. The Autotutor programmes, for example, included quite useful topics such as business management or office work or computer mathematics.

### Memory

Retrograde amnesia could be coped with, in the sense that old skills and routines could sometimes be relearnt. PTA could sometimes actually be of psychological benefit. Practical memory aids, practice in concentration and better initial registration of the facts to be remembered by using as many of the five senses as possible sometimes seemed to help, as did exercises in remembering and in the daily repetition and overlearning of important basic facts and skills. Nevertheless, the problem remained that where short-term memory was poor, then the ability to learn was poor and rehabilitation was slow.

REFERENCES

Russell G M 1975 An education therapist at work. RAF Education Bulletin no 12 autumn: 63-69
Russell G M 1978 An education therapist in the services. Therapy August: 6
Vivash E P 1972 The role of the training squadron at the Joint Services Medical Rehabilitation Unit. RAF Education Bulletin no 9 autumn: 13-17
Vivash E P 1973 Assessment and re-education at the JSMRU Services Education no 1 autumn: 8-11

# 6

# Physiotherapy: assessment and treatment of disordered motor function

'The brain understands movement not muscles'

## INTRODUCTION

The physical problems resulting from head injury are very varied and may present as any combination of the following: spasticity, rigidity, cerebellar incoordination, and dyspraxia. The picture may be further complicated by additional injuries such as fractures, dislocations and nerve lesions sustained at the time of the accident. Sensory disorders and perceptual problems will also affect motor performance. Prolonged unconsciousness and the necessity for surgery may delay the patient's admission to the rehabilitation centre, by which time contractures and abnormal movement patterns are often well established. A common sight is that of an incontinent, wheelchair-bound patient, whose motor performance is limited to a few abnormal and functionless patterns of movement.

The assessment of motor problems following head injury is complicated because it is likely that the motor function of the body will be affected as a whole unit. More emphasis must be placed upon the observation and analysis of patterns of movement rather than upon the measurement of individual joint range and muscle strength. 'The patient with spasticity is not too "weak" to move. The apparent weakness of muscles may not be real weakness but relative to the opposition of spastic antagonists' (Bobath 1969). Thus the resulting measurement of muscle strength has no value since it will vary according to any factors which may influence tone, for example, position of the patient, anxiety, environmental temperature. It is also extremely difficult to isolate one component in order to assess its severity or the contribution that it makes to the resulting abnormal movement. This is particularly true of spasticity, the predominant feature of physical problems in the head-injured patient.

In order to appreciate deviations from normal, an adequate understanding of both motor performance and development of movement in the normal individual is required. The term normal movement covers a wide spectrum. Motor performance will vary from one individual to another, for example, two people may use different methods to roll over or to get up from the floor. Even within the same individual variations occur: it is often found that coordination in the dominant hand is more precise than that in the non-dominant hand. Some people can achieve a more sophisticated level of coordination at certain skills than others, for example, musicians and sportsmen. However, normal motor function in all individuals still relies fundamentally on the presence of a basic framework of control of movement which is built up during the early years of development.

Although it is common knowledge that children develop in different ways and at different rates, for example, not all children crawl, nor do they all walk at the age of one year, there are still essential stages in the developmental sequence that must always be achieved. Head control must be established before eye focus is possible, postural stability of the shoulder girdle is necessary to allow the hands to be brought together in the midline, and the hands are only free to develop skilled activity when proximal postural stability is established. Balance in standing must be achieved before independent walking is possible. Thus an essential framework is being built up within all the recognisable variations and by the time full development of motor control has occurred an enormous variety of movement is at the disposal of the individual and can be used in many ways. The more frequently a particular movement is repeated the more efficient is its performance, until eventually, after continued repetition, a certain number of actions become automatic and are characteristic of the individual. He will have many more additional actions at his disposal, but as these are less well-rehearsed they are likely to be less efficiently performed.

The patients under discussion do not have this infinite variety of movement available to them. Disorders of tone and contractures of muscles and joints will dictate the basic posture and the manner in which movement can occur, and these predominantly abnormal influences will tend to be constant. The resulting movement from this abnormal posture must, of necessity, also be abnormal. Additionally, where spasticity is the predominant problem, the effort involved in preparing for a movement will of itself increase the spasticity. Thus the result of this will be that a limited number of activities are constantly produced in the wrong way and the more times they are repeated the more likely are they to become the learned automatic response.

However, in spite of an immensely varied and complex set of problems presented by the patient, it is possible to approach assessment in a logical and structured way.

## ASSESSMENT

### General impression
In order give a general picture of the level of independence, the therapist should place the patient in one of the following categories:

a. Walking independently, inside and outside
b. Walking with aids, inside and outside
c. Walking with aids, inside only
d. Confined to a wheelchair, but independent
e. Confined to a wheelchair, and dependent

Next, the postural abnormalities of each patient should be described. The set of problems listed below is an example of a typical pattern of sitting posture which may develop where there are alterations of tone.

'Poking' chin
Kyphosed thoracic spine
Reduced lumbar curve
Hips in insufficient flexion, although flexion may at first appear to predominate
A tendency to extension of the knees
Plantarflexed feet

Asymmetry will always be present, and the influence of this at the various levels should be noted. Detailed observation of the development of these patterns during the acute stage is needed in order that the underlying reasons for their origin can be investigated.

### Observation of movement
Initially, observation should be made of the movements the patient is able to achieve. Then the therapist should analyse the method used by the patient in completing each movement. In order to make this analysis the following points should be established.

Is the required movement possible?
If it can be achieved, is it performed normally or abnormally?
If it is abnormal, how does it differ from the normal?
With handling from the therapist, is it possible either to facilitate a movement previously impossible or to improve the quality of the abnormal movement?

| NAME | DATE |
|---|---|
| LOCOMOTOR ABILITY | SCORE 1 or 0 |
| Supine to prone over right | |
| Supine to prone over left | |
| Prone to supine over right | |
| Prone to supine over left | |
| Prone lying with elbow support | |
| Prone lying elbow support R | |
| Prone lying elbow support L | |
| Bridging | |
| Bridging moving to right | |
| Bridging moving to left | |
| Bridging moving up | |
| Bridging moving down | |
| Sits in long sitting | |
| Gets to long sitting | |
| Sitting | |
| Sitting moving to right | |
| Sitting moving to left | |
| Transfer right | |
| Transfer left | |
| Side sitting right | |
| Side sitting left | |
| Gets to side sitting right | |
| Gets to side sitting left | |
| Prone kneeling | |
| Gets to prone kneeling | |
| Crawling | |
| High kneeling | |
| Gets to high kneeling | |
| Half stand kneeling right knee | |
| Half stand kneeling left knee | |
| Gets to half stand kneeling right knee | |
| Gets to half stand kneeling left knee | |
| Standing | |
| Gets to standing | |
| Stands on right leg | |
| Stands on left leg | |
| TOTAL OUT OF 36 | |

**Fig. 6.1**    Chart for assessment of locomotor ability.

This is an attempt to realise the potential of the patient and illustrates the difficulty of dividing assessment and treatment: as soon as the patient is asked to move or is handled, it could be said that treatment has begun.

## Quantified assessment

### Locomotor function

Figure 6.1 shows the 36 progressions of movement, based on the normal developmental sequence. Starting at the top of the scale with rolling, and working down in order, the patient is asked to perform each movement in turn. Demonstration is given if the request is not fully understood. The patient scores one point for each movement he achieves unassisted, and zero if he fails. Originally half scores could be given as well, but these proved to be unreliable and were discarded. Specific instruction to therapists in the administration of the test is given, for example, when rolling, the patient must succeed by the third attempt, and when weight-bearing on one leg the position must be maintained for three seconds. As this is an achievement scale, it is possible for a patient to score 36 and yet still show abnormality of movement. The deficit in quality of movement will, in fact, be demonstrated either in the following test or on videotape. Wherever the quality of the movement is in doubt, the assessment is videotaped for subsequent analysis.

### Assessment of the dynamic interference by abnormalities of tone

Experience had shown that in the majority of patients control of movement returned proximally before distally, and that the degree of control could be influenced by the position of the body and head. In this part of the assessment each limb is examined in turn working from proximal to distal, with the patient in lying, prone lying, sitting and finally standing positions. When the level of control is determined, the movement is graded using a 0–5 scale, the more distal the control of movement the higher the grade given, 5 being normal. Figure 6.2 shows the criteria used and the positions for assessment. Again, it is important to record on videotape any deficit in quality or speed of movement. When distal control is present, though not considered to be normal, the patient is asked to repeat a number of finely coordinated movements, and the film of this performance will be compared later with subsequent assessments. Spasticity is not necessarily solely responsible for the alteration in the quality of movement: head injury will produce a mixture of lesions.

|  | R.ARM | L.ARM | R.LEG | L.LEG |
|---|---|---|---|---|
| Lying |  |  |  |  |
| Lying head to right |  |  |  |  |
| Lying head to left |  |  |  |  |
| Prone lying |  |  |  |  |
| Sitting |  |  |  |  |
| Standing |  |  |  |  |
| Standing head to right |  |  |  |  |
| Standing head to left |  |  |  |  |

SCALE OF GRADING

0 = Movement in one total pattern only; ie total flexion or extension.

1 = Movement both in flexion and extension, with some control of proximal joint.

2 = As in one, plus independent movement in middle joint.

3 = As in two, plus independent movement in distal joints.

4 = Good independent movement in distal joints, with some evidence of mass action on re-inforcement.

5 = Normal.

**Fig. 6.2**  Chart and grading scale for assessment of the dynamic interference by abnormality of tone.

*Sensory loss*

It became apparent that patients with considerable sensory loss generally made a poorer recovery than those with lesser or no sensory problems. This indicated a need for detailed sensory assessment. As many patients were severely handicapped, both in comprehension and expression, the method of testing had to be easy to explain and to require only a minimal response. This part of the assessment is spread over several sessions, as the patient may have difficulty in sustaining the necessary amount of concentration for more than a few minutes at a time. In fact, some patients are unable to attempt the sensory assessment initially, as their concentration is limited to a few seconds only. However, an experienced physiotherapist should be able to gain some impression of the amount of sensory loss by the way in which the patient responds during treatment.

The importance of the precise assessment of cortical sensory loss has been emphasised by McCollough & Sarmiento (1970), and although they were concerned with hemiplegia their remarks are relevant to the head-injured patient. They found that a limb will not regain normal function if the sensation is impaired, and they stressed that proximal as well as distal joint position sense must be tested in order to be able to predict the final degree of recovery.

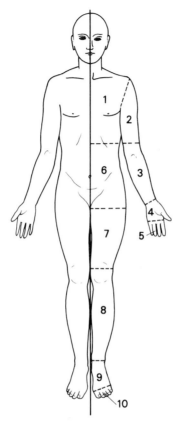

**Fig. 6.3**  Body diagram.

Figure 6.3 shows the body diagram on which the areas to be examined for superficial and deep sensation have been marked out. Sensation is tested from proximal to distal, using cotton wool for light touch and a blunt object such as the end of a pencil for deep sensation. Figure 6.4 shows the chart for recording and the scale of grading used. When examining joint position sense it is important to know whether the deficit is confined to the more distal joints or whether the more proximal joints are also involved. Many joints are examined, and the testing is performed from proximal to distal. Scoring is based on the scale of grading shown in Figure 6.5: the awareness of movement in each joint is recorded. The therapist demonstrates the method of testing to the patient before asking him to close his eyes. Localisation is tested in the hands only, and the accuracy of localisation in each area is recorded. Figure 6.6 shows the criteria used for scoring.

| | SUPERFICIAL | | DEEP | |
|---|---|---|---|---|
| | RIGHT | LEFT | RIGHT | LEFT |
| 1 | | | | |
| 2 | | | | |
| 3 | | | | |
| 4 | | | | |
| 5 | | | | |
| 6 | | | | |
| 7 | | | | |
| 8 | | | | |
| 9 | | | | |
| 10 | | | | |
| TOTAL | | | | |
| A | | | | |
| B | | | | |
| C | | | | |
| TOTAL | | | | |

SCALE OF GRADING

SUPERFICIAL

0 = Anaesthetic

1 = Hypoaesthetic

2 = Hyperaesthetic

3 = Normal

DEEP

0 = No awareness

1 = Partial awareness

2 = Full awareness

**Fig. 6.4** Chart and scale of grading for recording superficial and deep sensation.

|  | RIGHT | LEFT |
|---|---|---|
| Shoulders |  |  |
| Elbows |  |  |
| Wrists |  |  |
| MPs |  |  |
| IPs |  |  |
| Thumb MPs |  |  |
| Thumb IPs |  |  |
| Hips |  |  |
| Knees |  |  |
| Ankles |  |  |
| MIPs |  |  |

SCALE OF GRADING

0 = Unaware of movement

1 = Aware of extremes only

2 = Aware of gross movement, more than $60^{1}$

3 = Aware of coarse movement, more than $30^{1}$

4 = Aware of fine movements.

5 = Normal

**Fig. 6.5** Chart and scale of grading for joint position sense.

LOCALISATION

A = Palm   B = Fingers   C = Thumb

0 = Unaware

1 = Aware but out of area

2 = Aware and in area

3 = Aware to within one square inch

4 = Aware to within 1/4 square inch

5 = Normal

**Fig. 6.6** Criteria for establishing accuracy of localisation.

## Gait

A simple method for recording patterns of walking can be carried out by placing the patient's feet in talcum powder and measuring the resulting footprints, as shown in Figure 6.7. With the use of a ruler and a protractor, step length, dynamic base and foot angles can be measured.

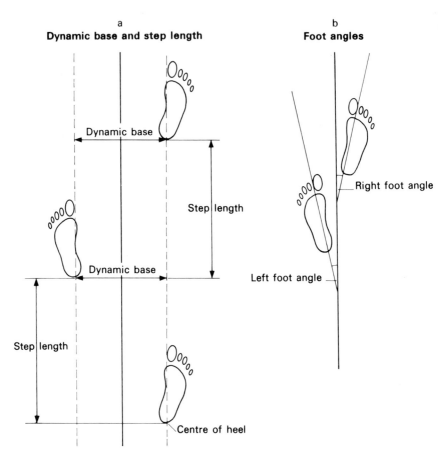

Fig. 6.7a & b   Method of recording gait by analysis of tread pattern.

## Dyspraxia

It was found that the textbook definition of dyspraxia did not cover all the manifestations of this problem as seen in head-injured patients. In fact, it was felt that the term 'sequencing disorders' was a more accurate definition. The principal difficulties arising from a sequencing problem are as follows:

a.  an inability to *conceptualise* the sequence required
b.  an inability to *initiate* the correct sequence
c.  an inability to perform the sequence in the correct *order*
d.  an inability to *change* from one sequence to another
e.  an inability to *interrupt* the sequence at will
f.  an inability to *alter* the speed of the sequence

Although these remarks pertain to movement, these problems may arise simultaneously in other areas, such as speech and thought. The existence of the problems can be difficult to establish, partly due to inadequate assessment techniques, but also due to a lack of recognition of their existence. However, a therapist with experience should be able to assess whether a patient's lack of performance arises from purely physical difficulties or whether the physical disabilities are in fact insufficiently severe to cause the low level of response exhibited. Furthermore, this group of patients show inconsistencies in their response. It appears from past experience that there are often ways of eliciting a correct response at an automatic level, but as soon as the patient's attention is drawn to the required movement there is difficulty in performing the movement.

*Case example*
Patient A, when asked to bend his elbow, was unable to do so, but when asked to look at his watch he then bent his elbow automatically. This variability of response can unfortunately be wrongly interpreted as lack of cooperation by the patient.

## Contractures
Unfortunately, these deformities are often found in patients referred to the rehabilitation centre, and the reason for their origin is not always clear, but it is considered likely that the following factors may contribute to their development:
a.  position of the patient during the unconscious stage
b.  severe and prolonged spasticity which may be further increased when pain and septic focus are present
c.  associated injuries which may make undesirable positioning inevitable
d.  associated injuries which may themselves lead to contractures, e.g. fractures or dislocations

The possibility of the presence of ectopic calcification must not be overlooked, and any suspect joints should be radiographed. The joints most susceptible to this problem are elbows, hips and spine.

When examining a contracted joint in the presence of spasticity, the therapist may find that after inhibition of the spasticity the contracture is in fact far less severe than was at first thought. However, in some cases the contracture will be found to be almost entirely due to shortening of soft tissue. The problem can then be isolated to a particular muscle group by testing in various positions, e.g. if the affected foot is held in plantarflexion, then testing for the degree of contracture should be performed with the knee in both flexion and extension in order to determine whether or not the gastrocnemius muscle is involved.

### Peripheral nerve lesions

These injuries may be sustained at the time of the accident, e.g. a brachial plexus or ulnar nerve lesion. They may also result from prolonged pressure during the unconscious stage, and an example of this is pressure over the elbow causing ulnar lesions. When the patients are severely disabled, a peripheral nerve lesion may escape notice at first, but later it may be recognised as areas of specific muscle wasting become apparent, accompanied by an appropriate sensory loss. Finally, when the patient begins to move, a typical deformity may be observed.

## PLANNING THE TREATMENT PROGRAMME

When all these assessments have been completed, the motor ability of the patient can be seen but this should not be considered to be a complete picture until the assessments from all the departments involved have been combined to give a profile of the disabilities of the patient. No one assessment should be considered in isolation.

The results of the assessments are discussed at the weekly clinical meetings of the therapeutic staff, and the treatment programme for each new patient is devised. Initially some patients will be unable to cope with a full programme, but treatment may be increased as their tolerance increases. Although some patients have multiple handicaps it may be necessary to emphasise the treatment for one problem at a time. For instance, it is essential that a very immobile patient learns to transfer as soon as possible, thus a large part of the day may be spent on this teaching in various practical situations, whereas for another patient the priorities may be entirely different.

*Case example*
Patient B had a severe memory disorder and needed initially to form a relationship with a limited number of people. Although there were some physical problems present, the initial memory retraining took precedence.

# TREATMENT

During discussion of treatment emphasis will be placed on the more severely physically disabled patients. The two most important considerations at this stage are firstly that the patient is extremely immobile, and secondly that any available movements are likely to be in abnormal patterns. Every time an abnormal pattern is used, it becomes reinforced, and as there is a limited choice of movement available these abnormal movements will become quickly learned.

First, the therapist should ensure that if the patient is confined to a wheelchair, then it is of the correct size and type. If the posture is asymmetrical, the sensory input will be asymmetrical, and this 'uneven' input through weight-bearing surfaces will begin to feel normal to the patient: when this is corrected the more symmetrical posture will feel 'wrong' or uncomfortable.

As has been stated already most patients exhibit a mixture of problems, but for clarity each problem and its treatment will be dealt with separately. It will be rare for any of these problems to occur in isolation.

## Spasticity

Spasticity is the most common of all the physical problems and the one which promotes the most discussion. In order that the patient is able to achieve a more normal movement, and have more variety of movement, then the spasticity must first be inhibited. This should not be considered as a separate part of treatment, but must be accompanied by and associated with movement. A static approach to treatment must be avoided at all times. Initially it may be necessary for the therapist to use facilitation techniques which will elicit normal automatic motor responses. This stage should be viewed as part of the progression towards voluntary movement — gradually the control is handed over to the patient, until eventually it is hoped that he will be able to initiate and carry out the movement independently and in a more normal pattern.

In order to be able to re-educate movement in a logical way, it is necessary to re-establish the more basic and proximal movements first, with an emphasis on head control. The locomotor sequence, described earlier, can be used as a guide for progression of movement, but the sequence must not be rigidly adhered to: there is no question of a patient achieving a movement perfectly before being allowed to attempt a more complicated movement. In addition, the sequence can be used as a means of relating early movements to later movements.

The emphasis for a particular treatment session may be upon early mat activities, but the relevance of these movements must be shown to the patient by working from rolling into sitting or standing positions. The reason behind the importance of achieving this basic framework arises from observations that patients can improve their walking pattern not necessarily by practising walking, but by building up the earlier activities.

A recent innovation for the treatment of spasticity has been the introduction of mobile, inflatable equipment, as shown in Figures 6.8 and 6.9. It has been found that the use of this equipment leads to the release of spasticity and the facilitation of automatic postural reactions, thus renewing the patient's acquaintance with experiences of movement of which he has been deprived for some time. When the mattress is used, there is a more even distribution of weight than when the patient is placed on a flat mat area, thus the sensory input is not confined to a few bony points, and a greater surface of the body is in contact with the mattress. The patient has a feeling of comfort, and this will be another factor in decrease of the spasticity. When lying on a mat, there is continual emphasis of uncomfortable sensory input through the same small areas, whereas the use of the mattress enlarges and alters the areas of sensory input. The equipment provides an unstable surface for the patient: merely lying over the beach ball will demand some degree of postural adjustment, and this in turn will be another significant factor in the reduction of spasticity. The mobile equipment can be used in a variety of ways and adapted to suit the individual needs of each patient. Figures 6.8 and 6.9 illustrate the use of the mattress and the ball in two different cases. As the mobility of the patient increases and more voluntary control is gained, more advanced activities can be attempted (Figs. 6.10 and 6.11). If spasticity is significantly reduced by the use of this apparatus, then this form of treatment may be used as a preliminary to standing and walking activities.

The tilt table has been found to be highly beneficial for patients who are unable to stand or be stood due to severe flexor spasticity (Fig. 6.12). However, as soon as the patient has some degree of control in this position, the use of the tilt table should be gradually phased out. It is essential that the patient weight-bears and develops control in an antigravity position as early as possible, although walking at this stage is not considered to be either practical or desirable. Care should be taken to ensure that weight is taken through the heels and that it is evenly distributed.

Spasticity may affect facial movements, breathing, chewing and

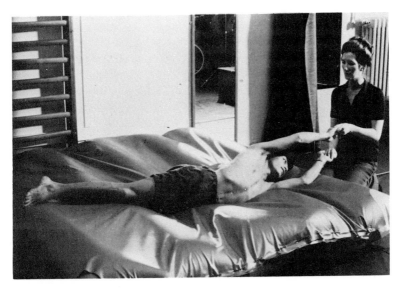

**Fig. 6.8** Use of inflatable mattress to reduce spasticity.

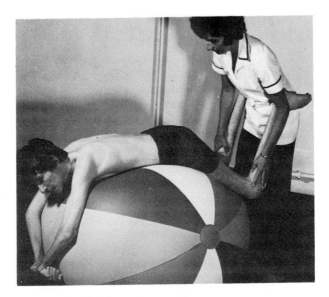

**Fig. 6.9** Use of inflatable ball to reduce spasticity.

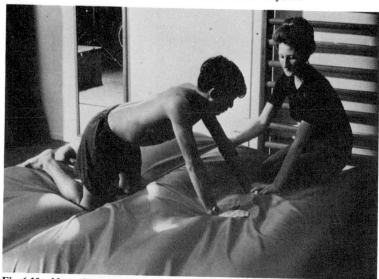

**Fig. 6.10**    More advanced exercise using inflatable mattress.

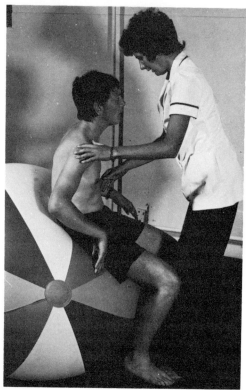

**Fig. 6.11**    More advanced exercise using inflatable ball.

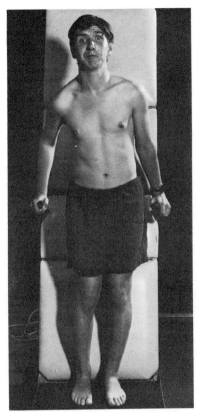

**Fig. 6.12**    A tilt table can be useful for patients unable to stand due to severe flexor spasticity.

swallowing. As an adequate control of these movements is necessary for speech production, it is profitable if the physiotherapist and speech therapist can work together for the reduction of spasticity and a more normal motor response. In these cases, the techniques of brushing and icing developed by Miss Rood can be used, with discretion. The area to be brushed or iced is always very specific, and the likely effect upon myotomes and dermatomes needs to be known. Also, the effect of the application may in some cases be central, for example, brushing the skin of the ear and the outer one-third of the forehead has a central inhibitory effect, whereas icing the lips and tongue has the opposite effect. In fact, these particular techniques form only a small part of a wide concept of treatment for many different neurological problems. The aim is always to obtain as normal a response as possible by applying the appropriate afferent stimuli. Conscious cortical control by the patient is not needed.

## Cerebellar incoordination

In general, cerebellar problems are difficult to treat. The cerebellar patient, unlike the spastic patients, does have the full range of movements available but with no control. Patients with this problem lack proximal fixation and this manifests itself in a lack of distal coordination. Treatment should be directed towards improving the proximal stability before concentrating on the distal problems. It may be found that as the proximal control improves, the distal incoordination is less severe than was at first thought.

Emphasis on weight-bearing activities is essential in order to obtain the necessary co-contraction. In addition, techniques of tapping may be applied by the therapist, though these should be used with great care where there are additional problems of spasticity as tapping will increase tone. Care should also be taken to avoid a static position for the patient while weight-bearing activities are being taught. Mobility within the stability is the aim, the accent being on patterns of movement rather than upon static positions. Controlled movement is achieved only when there is a combination of mobility and stability.

Using weighted aids has been found to be helpful in some cases of cerebellar incoordination, such as poor head control causing feeding problems, for which a weighted cap can be worn by the patient during meal times. A weighted waistcoat can be worn for ataxic problems in walking (Fig. 6.13). Alternatively weighted shoes may be used. There may be occasions when weights on the wrists are beneficial. It should be noted when using weights that consideration must be given to the quantity of weight added. For example, a weighted skull-cap may contain as little as half a pound of lead shot, whereas a weighted jacket could carry as much as 10 pounds. Each patient must be assessed individually in order to establish the degree of weighting necessary to control the incoordination, and the use of central weighting should be limited to those who are able to maintain a reasonably symmetrical posture. There is some evidence to suggest that the continued use of weighted aids causes the patient to adjust to their effect, thus reducing their benefit. Therefore their use should perhaps be limited to the times of day when they are most required, rather than being worn continuously.

## Dyspraxia

Dyspraxic patients need to be able to produce a consistent and correct response both automatically and voluntarily. Treatment must aim to tackle one sequence of movements at a time. Initially constant repetition of a particular sequence is demanded of the patient in one

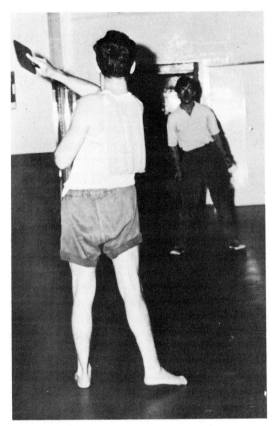

Fig. 6.13   Use of a weighted waistcoat may help general activity level.

situation only, with as much physical and verbal help as is necessary
from the therapist. Eventually the patient is expected to produce the
sequence of movement at will as well as spontaneously, and in any
situation. He should also be able to interrupt the sequence or alter its
speed. In cases where the patient has an inability to visualise the
required movement, the therapist must either demonstrate or use
other visual aids such as video. Verbal reinforcement may be helpful,
but if used it should be carefully selected with the help of the speech
therapist and used consistently. It is very important that sufficient
reinforcement and facilitation is given to allow the patient to succeed
in his task. It has been suggested that this group of patients are
generally difficult to treat, but this has not been the experience at this
centre. In fact some of the patients who have made the most dramatic
improvements have been in this category.

## Contractures

Less severe contractures involving the soft tissues will normally respond quickly to a dynamic programme of re-education of movement. Weight-bearing through the lower limbs is essential to reduce flexed knees and hips and to promote dorsiflexion of the feet: this can be initiated in the early stages by the use of a tilt table. Care should be taken to ensure that the heels are in contact with the floor or platform, for if weight is taken through the toes then the extensor thrust is accentuated. Minor contractures may present no problem to the advancement of the motor function of the patient, but more severe contractures may seriously impede further physical progress, and where this is the case an alternative approach may be needed. One method which has been used for these cases has been the use of serial plaster cylinders. Ankles, knees, interphalangeal joints and wrists have all responded well to this regime.

Ideally a plaster cylinder should be applied only when the tissues surrounding the affected joint are relaxed, in order that maximal reduction of the contracture is obtained, and it may be necessary therefore to apply ice or otherwise to inhibit spasticity prior to the application. Plenty of padding is used under the plaster, paying special attention to bony areas, or areas of sensory loss.

Knees and ankles are generally encased in plaster for approximately ten days. A few days after the initial application, the plaster may be cut and 'wedged' further open in order to produce more of a stretch on the contracted joint. When the plaster is removed a decrease in the extent of the contracture is frequently found. If the contracture is very severe, then a series of stretch plasters may be necessary. During the period of immobilisation functional activities are continued whenever possible (Fig. 6.14). It is essential that weight-bearing is emphasised for the patients wearing lower limb plasters. The procedure for applying plasters to interphalangeal joints differs in that the plaster is left remaining on the finger for a maximum of two days. It is important to note that the contractures associated with ectopic calcification need careful handling: in the acute stage the condition can be exacerbated by any stretch on the soft tissues surrounding the joint, so stretch plasters are contraindicated.

## Surgery

With severe fracture dislocation of the head of femur a joint replacement may be necessary, and surgery may be considered for removal of gross ectopic calcification, but the indications are not precise. Surgery may be suggested for some soft tissue lesions, but it is well worth attempting the procedures already described first. The

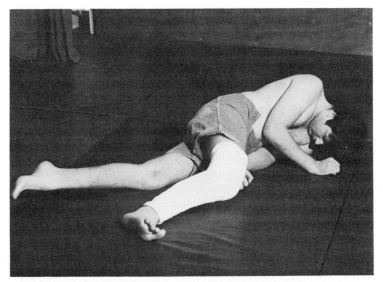

**Fig. 6.14**  Patient performing mat activities while still in plaster cast.

long-term implications of surgical intervention need to be considered, for example, after tendon lengthening of the hamstrings some patients will experience difficulty in activities such as standing up and sitting down. These complications may eventually present more of a problem than the original contracture. Tenotomy of the tendo Achilles can sometimes lead to a general decrease in spasticity.

**Nerve lesions**
Normally the treatment of these lesions can be incorporated quite successfully into the programme of re-education of movement. Where there has been sensory loss, then sensory re-education must be attempted as soon as recovery commences. The therapist should note the development of any typical deformity, and a decision will have to be made on the need for a splint. The complication of other factors such as spasticity may mean that the introduction of a lively splint would be impractical.

**Sensory disorders**
General treatment is directed towards an attempt to provide the correct sensory input in order to gain a response. The emphasis now is directed towards patients who show a marked loss of sensation or proprioception.

It has been said that 'a fundamental precept for normal sensation is movement' (Wynn Parry & Salter 1976). When watching a person exploring an object in order to assess its texture, weight, shape and temperature, it can be seen that unless motor control is present, the sensory information cannot be interpreted accurately. Thus, when attempting to re-educate sensory disorders it is important that, whenever possible, motor participation is demanded of the patient. For the patient with severe sensory problems and minimal movement, who is unable to alter or increase his sensory input in any way, the aim of the therapist must be to help the patient to experience a greater variety of sensation through weight-bearing and movement. The mobile equipment described earlier is considered to be extremely useful for this purpose. When using the mattress or the beach ball, sensory input can be introduced through a larger area of the body than when the patient is being treated on a mat, and in a greater variety of ways. The unstable surface of the equipment ensures that sensation and movement are experienced simultaneously.

When there is a return of some sensation and control of movement distally, then sensory retraining can commence. A similar pattern is followed to that which has been devised for sensory loss following peripheral nerve lesions (Salter 1970). With the eyes closed the patient is asked to discriminate between blocks of different size, shape and weight, then to describe different textures and finally to name everyday objects. In order to retrain this sense the patient spends part of the session with his eyes open using visual reinforcement. In order to be able to succeed in this part of the treatment the patient must have some awareness of superficial sensation.

In this chapter an attempt has been made to describe the physiotherapy approach to the treatment of disordered motor function. However, it must be appreciated that physiotherapists do not work in isolation, and that a combined therapy approach is adopted whenever possible. A close working relationship with the nursing staff is also essential in order that activities taught in the department during the day, can be reinforced by the nurses on the wards.

REFERENCES

Bobath B 1969 The treatment of neuromuscular disorders by improving patterns of coordination. Physiotherapy 55: 18-22
Bobath B, Bobath K 1975 Motor development in the different types of cerebral palsy. Heinemann, London
Evans C D et al 1976 Rehabilitation of the brain-damaged survivor. Injury 8: 80
Goff B 1972 The application of recent advances in neurophysiology to Miss M Rood's concept of neuromuscular facilitation. Physiotherapy 58: 409-415
Goff B 1976 Grading of spasticity and its effect on voluntary movement. Physiotherapy 62: 358
Graham O 1975 Closed circuit television assessment of disability following severe head injury. Physiotherapy 61: 272

McCullough N C, Sarmiento A 1970 Functional prognosis of the hemiplegic. Journal of the Florida Medical Association 57: 31-34

Newcombe F 1975 Recovery curves in acquired dyslexia. Journal of Neurological Science 24: 127-133

Salter M I 1970 Sensory re-education of the hand. Progress in Physical Therapy 1, no 3

Scrutton D S, Robson P 1968 The gait of 50 normal children. Physiotherapy

Stichbury J C 1975 Assessment of disability following severe head injury. Physiotherapy 61: 268

Stichbury J C, Davenport M J, Middleton F R I 1980 Head-injured patients — a combined therapeutic approach. Physiotherapy 66: 288-292

Wynn Parry C B, Salter M I 1976 Sensory re-education after median nerve lesions. The Hand 8: 250-257

# 7

# Occupational therapy

## INTRODUCTION

Many brain-damaged patients have to leave the acute hospital long before they are socially independent or ready to return to work. Among them are some who would benefit from attending a rehabilitation centre where they could be given treatment which, it is believed, will help them to effect the maximum independence, socially and financially. Recovery from head injury can take many months or years so that it is not possible for the patient to spend all of this period in a rehabilitation centre, neither is it desirable. It is not yet clear, however, what alternative patterns can be presented. It may be better for several admissions to be spread over a period of years, interspersed with attempts at resettlement within the community. Much will depend upon the whole needs of the patient and also the availability of other facilities and suitability or otherwise of the home situation.

As with the other medical and paramedical disciplines, much of the advice given is apocryphal and didactic and many different packages of rehabilitation are designed, none of which yet have been evaluated effectively, though some recent experience at Northwick Park, albeit concerned with stroke cases, gives some encouragement that a more constructive approach may be taken in the future.

In the occupational therapy department it is the aim of the therapists to produce methods of evaluation and treatment which will specifically identify perceptual problems and also make a practical evaluation of the limitations of physical ability in the performance of activities of daily living: and finally to produce therapy programmes which will help the patient overcome either or both of these problems. It is considered most important to make the therapy programmes relevant to the patient, not beneath his competence and dignity, nor too difficult to be attempted successfully.

## ASSESSMENT

The initial assessment in a rehabilitation centre should be made during a period of not less than two to three weeks, particularly with the more handicapped patients. This is because the patient may be disturbed by the move to a strange environment so that the initial performance is significantly lower than it was on the discharge from hospital. Also, head-injured patients often tire quickly so that the amount achieved each session before performance is affected by fatigue may be significantly limited. In the occupational therapy department, the following factors are assessed, though the emphasis on each will depend on the other departments' repertoire of assessment: physical ability, the identification of perceptual and intellectual deficit, the recognition of communication problems, the level of social independence — especially in activities of daily living — and finally early retraining in old skills or advice as to new avenues for exploration if the handicap will prevent the patients going back to their original jobs. It may be that all of these factors will contribute to the handicap, or that one will predominate. The initial aim of the treatment will also be modified by subsequent progress so that priorities will change, and therefore it is essential that the treatment team work together, communicating any changes that take place, and altering the patient's programme in accordance with his changing abilities.

From a perusal of the list of the basic series of assessments it will be apparent that there is substantial opportunity for overlap with the work done in other departments. Consequently coordination and integration to avoid useless overlap is of prime importance. This re-emphasises the importance of establishing effective and practical working relationships between departments.

## Physical assessment
It may be necessary for the occupational therapist to carry out only a superficial physical assessment since the physiotherapy department will normally be doing this in depth. But the occupational therapist's assessment needs to be sufficient to judge the level of suitable activities to be provided.

### Truncal stability
The patient should be assessed seated straight upright in a chair. In the early stages support may be necessary. A long mirror in front of the patient may be helpful in some cases so they can get feedback from this as to their position. Positioning of the limbs may help to maintain trunk posture and this will also help in the early functional assessment.

### Lower limbs
The feasibility of transferring a patient from wheelchair to an ordinary upright chair or to a toilet should be done as soon as possible. Walking patterns, if practicable, are best decided in conjunction with physiotherapy but once established should be practised consistently

by all departments. Activities in the occupational therapy department can also be chosen to encourage standing tolerance and balance. Care should be taken, especially in the early stages of rehabilitation, to monitor the programme so as not to overtire the patient or introduce conflicting aspects of the programme.

*Upper limbs*

The occupational therapist should start the assessment with a physical examination of the upper limbs so that she car decide whether lack of success is due to loss of physical movement, e.g. from fracture, or to other causes, i.e. perceptual. Again this should be related to other initial medical and paramedical assessments. The prime movements to be assessed are those of the scapula and shoulder girdle, the flexion and extension of the elbow, pronation and supination of forearm, flexion and extension of wrists and fingers, and finally, practical manual dexterity.

The treatment of head-injured patients may initially have to be directed more towards physical disability as it is often difficult for them to appreciate or to accept any reason other than a physical one for their inability to perform tasks successfully. It is therefore important to have a selection of activities which in fact serve a dual role, such as tasks which involve finger movement but also which may help to demonstrate and identify spatial problems.

**Perceptual and intellectual assessment**

It is a sad fact of life that many rehabilitation centres lack the services of a clinical psychologist. Consequently the task of assessing the perceptual, intellectual and emotional aspects of the patient's problems may fall into the ambit of the occupational therapy department. Where a clinical psychologist is available, as at Rivermead Rehabilitation Centre, then many of the following tasks will be undertaken by that department. Recent collaboration between the British Association of Occupational Therapists and the British Psychological Society has allowed a limited battery of tests to be performed by occupational therapists and this provides an extremely helpful adjunct for many departments. It is even more rare for there to be sufficient clinical psychologists available to give treatment, so this too will often become the responsibility of the occupational therapy as well as other departments.

*Perceptual dysfunction*

It is comparatively easy to see and assess the patient's physical disability, but much more difficult to define perceptual dysfunction (Figs 7.1 and 7.2). In order to understand normal behaviour, the methods by which skills are acquired during infancy and early

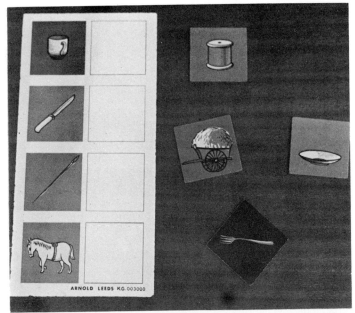

**Fig. 7.1**   Having found that the patient can recognise objects — can he now match things which go together? This is a useful activity when speech is absent.

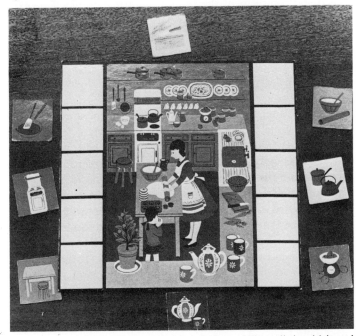

**Fig. 7.2**   A more complicated picture which again shows ability to distinguish items in a picture. Form constancy problems may become apparent through inability to recognise items produced differently, e.g. the frying pan and egg slice.

childhood which enable adults to react appropriately and to live in the environment, must be understood, since some of the treatment programmes will have to go over already learned material.

Information from outside the body is received through the five senses, sight, sound, hearing, touch and taste. For each of these senses there has to be a conversion of energy from that which is present in the environment to that which can be perceived. For example, radiation within the physical spectrum of light can only be perceived if the transducing apparatus, i.e. the eye and the optic tracts, are intact. No visual information about the environment inside a blindfold will be gained (though developments of techniques of sensory substitution and the phenomena of blind sight cast some doubts even on this). It is important first to establish the integrity of the five basic senses, though with least emphasis placed on that of taste and smell, unless the occupation of the patient makes it crucial.

*Sight*
Eighty per cent of perception is said to be derived through visual experience, and vision is used to augment other senses to a great degree. The reverse process is also true. For example, while listening to a person speaking, the lips of the speaker are frequently closely watched and complement the auditory information to a large extent, and this may be one of the reasons why some people dislike using the telephone. Specific disabilities may appear which should be identified through the initial medical, but the impact may not be fully appreciated on the ability of the patient until the detailed examination is done in the department. Any or all of the following may be identified.

*Hemianopia* interferes with receiving the correct stimulus because only half the visual field, be it to the left or to the right, is available for vision. The anatomy of this has been described earlier and the implications as to whether the dominant or non-dominant hemisphere is involved and the portion of the optic tract involved has also been discussed. Similarly the phenomenon of 'blind sight' in an hemianopic field is discussed in a later chapter on new developments, but for the moment in the OT department it is of practical importance to be sure of whether information is visually received from right or left or both. Hemianopia may be either homonomous, i.e. totally to the left or to the right, or may involve either the nasal or the temporal aspects of the field, i.e. the patient will be unable to see either to the sides or to the middle. The macula where most of the vision is concentrated may be spared in either event, in which case the effective handicap can be substantially lessened.

*Diplopia* may affect the patient in that two images which are not fused are formed. In addition to the fact that this condition may be associated with other problems of incoordination, double vision is in itself confusing, particularly if one image is not quite parallel either vertically or horizontally to the other. This can be practically treated in a physiotherapy or occupational therapy department simply by occluding with a patch one eye or the other, though it is important to ensure that one eye is not occluded by itself at the expense of the other permanently, for otherwise the perception of vision through the affected eye may eventually diminish, leaving a person essentially amblyopic, as with a childhood squint.

## Visual perception

Defects of visual perception mainly occur with patients who have a left cerebral lesion. They can be subdivided.

*Figure ground discrimination.* This is the ability to focus attention on any one object and abstract it from other objects surrounding it (Fig. 7.3). The patient's attention tends to jump from one object to another so that here the amount of material presented is very important. If the patient is shown a multiple picture, he is unable to pick out the one object required.

*Form constancy or perceptual constancy.* This is the ability to recognise known objects if they are placed at unfamiliar angles or are of different size, colour or thickness. Or, if for any other reason, the two identical objects are not presented in exactly the same way, they may not be recognised as similar.

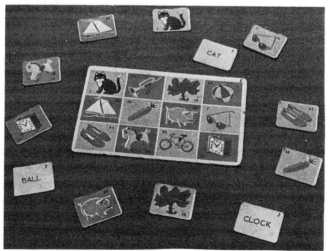

**Fig. 7.3**   Figure-ground discrimination made easy by having each item shown in its own frame.

*Activities*

Matching pictures where each object is individually framed; it is much more difficult to pick out objects in a complex picture. The patient may have particular difficulty with items which are not identically reproduced, which shows constancy problems.

Activities can be related to practical daily activities. Can he recognise his garments? Can she recognise the things she needs in the kitchen? Can he sort coins?

*Reasoning* can only come after the patient is able to interpret what he is looking at. It may be further hindered by receptive or expressive dysphasia. An early test for reasoning ability involves matching pairs, e.g. knife and fork.

## Problems generally connected with damage to the right hemisphere

These include loss of body image, appreciation of self in space and spatial relations of objects in space.

The patient may have a poor concept of body image. He may not be able to name parts of his body or manipulate his limbs in space. He may become confused with right and left and not really know where he is in space. This can be further exacerbated by sensory problems. He may have difficulty crossing the mid-line (we all know the patient who only shaves or combs his hair on one side). These difficulties will be made worse if the patient has sensory loss on one side or he has a homonymous hemionopia.

*Activities*

Labelling parts of the body on a picture or, better still, using his own body. The practical activity of dressing when the patient is usually well motivated because of his wish to achieve this independence, is usually very beneficial. Putting pegs or shapes into holes, joining dots, putting together things such as a simple wooden jigsaw where he must oppose the piece in order to succeed.

*Inattention*

Some of these patients may only have lost their appreciation of spatial relationships. Others may be further disabled by a complete or partial loss of appreciation of the presence of their left side. This is usually known as left-sided inattention, neglect or denial. It is sometimes seen on the right but is much less common. The patient is often quite unaware of his problem. If he is aware he may still be quite unable to do anything about it. He cannot reason or think logically about anything to the left of the midline. He may have lost the ability to sift and sort logically and is hindered by perseveration. A patient may appear perfectly normal in conversation, but when faced with a simple written problem he will read the right half only and still come up with an answer. He may read only half of a word or a number and not realise this cannot be right. He may also only see the right half or things placed on his right. His memory may appear defective and he may be disorientated because he is not receiving all the necessary information. In fact, the patient is no longer able to function as a 'whole person'.

*Sound*
Sound may be distorted for a variety of very simple reasons. Some of them will be identified within the other examinations but it is important that the occupational therapist knows whether there is deafness present, which is the side that she has to speak from and whether in fact the hearing impairment is so severe that other visual forms of communication may have to be used. It is also possible that hearing may be distorted so that although words and sounds can be heard they do not appear normal.

*Touch*
Sensibility of any or all modalities may also be lost. From the therapist's point of view, it is essential to know whether the ability to perceive and respond appropriately to pain is still present. If not, particular precautions have to be taken in order to ensure that no activity exercise can expose the patient to extremes of temperature or to sharp edges which, because of altered sensation, he will have to guard against. Similarly, loss of proprioception and altered stereognosis may make the performance of many tasks extremely difficult.

*Taste and smell*
Taste and smell are perceived by different portions of the brain. They also have different systems of transduction. Taste strictly can identify only four sensations, these being salt, sweet, bitter and sour, and this information is mediated through various parts of the tongue to the brain. All other forms of what we frequently refer to as taste are in fact functions of the olfactory nerve and its portion of the brain, as can be readily witnessed by the loss of taste when anybody's nose is blocked by a cold. Nonetheless the loss of the sense of smell (amosmia) is a major disability and provides a severe handicap for a patient whose prime task may be the preparation of food and may also limit the abilities of a housewife in providing acceptable food since she cannot judge the taste.

*Memory*
The most important practical distinction to draw is that between the patient losing his memory traces from before the accident, which is unusual, but not necessarily devastating, to the loss of ability to acquire new information or to recall two items in succession — which is most disabling. Tests developed with the speech therapy department, and retraining programmes using any available clues should be used.

*Speech and communication*
Speech and communication should be assessed closely with the speech therapy department.

## ACTIVITIES OF DAILY LIVING

Social independence is probably the most important factor in planning future prospects for the patient. The strain put upon families by a totally dependent member may well prove intolerable. The degree of independence required of individuals before they can return home depends on their home situation so that the aims of the therapist will be somewhat dependent on this factor. For instance, the patient who lives alone will generally need more independence and the time at which he can go home will depend on this and upon the amount of help available from the community.

With head-injured patients it is often factors such as a slowness to take initiative and accept responsibility which affect their ability to become independent. Relatives are frequently overprotective because of the patient's reluctance to manage for himself. It is, therefore, most important for the patient to have adequate practice before going home so that he builds up some ability and confidence. It is then equally important that the relatives are shown what the patient can do and how they should help if this is necessary. It may then be necessary to show the patient and the family how to manage in their own home surroundings.

Other factors which stand in the way of the patient becoming independent are poor memory, lack of motivation and insight. Patients with perceptual problems, spatial or inattention problems, apraxia or agnosia, may show these difficulties in activities of daily living although this is not necessarily so in all activities. Each patient has to be assessed on all activities which are necessary for him, and practice given in the areas in which he finds difficulty. ADL indices are produced widely, and have been reviewed by Donaldson. Whether they are used from derived sources, or designed on the unit, matters little, but the precepts already mentioned about assessments in general still hold good.

## FUTURE WORK PROSPECTS

Many months, or even years, may pass before the patient is ready to contemplate any type of work. It is obviously much easier for the housewife to return to her job as she can be considerably aided in her task by family, friends or other home help: a person returning to open employment must be able to cope adequately or suffer the severe setback of losing his job.

## MANAGEMENT

### General

It is a useful introduction for the patient to the department if the first task he is asked to do is to fill in a card with his name, address, occupation, hobbies and interests; and also to state if he has any particular problems of which he is aware. This will give the therapist valuable information so that she can then assess what a relevant level of treatment may be. For instance, at the most basic, it tells the therapist whether the patient can either read, write or copy. At a more sophisticated level, it may indicate a receptive loss, expressive loss or an inability to understand or express language. By the way the answers are written, there may be the first hint of inattention or spatial problems. Further information will of course be obtained by specific testing, but the initial introduction and the initial conversation may often provide important clues as to the way the rest of the examination should be conducted. It is also clear that a lot of the initial assessment will clarify what aspects of the handicap will receive priority. So that wherever hierarchal assessment shows up the handicap, so it indicates the level of treatment.

Patients in the early stages after head injury are very insecure and frightened. This state may show itself in various ways. The patient may appear aggressive. This aggressiveness may be as a result of cortical irritation or it may be a result of insecurity to which the patient over-reacts in self-defence. The therapist should be consistent, supportive and positive in her approach. Having found the patient's level of behaviour and achievement ability she should have consistent set limits which the patient learns he is expected to achieve. As with a child, this gives the patient a feeling of security.

Activities must be intellectually right and provide sufficient interest so that the patient can channel his emotions and achieve some goal,

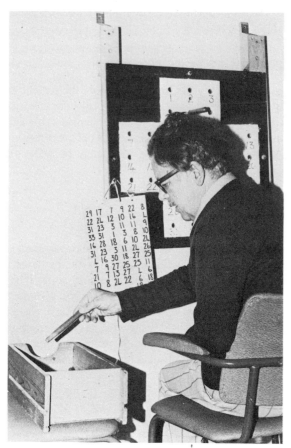

**Fig. 7.4** Solitaire is an extremely useful activity. Here the patient with a left hemiplegia is having his attention drawn to the left. By following the chart he should end up with one central peg.

however small (Figs 7.4 and 7.5). The patient should be adequately supervised so that if he has difficulties these can be noted and the patient can be helped to overcome them. This can be particularly important for patients with insight into their problems who find they are unable to perform basic tasks — which again can be a frightening experience.

Another important factor is the work atmosphere. This should be friendly and unruffled. With poor concentration and feelings of insecurity these patients are often easily distracted by their surroundings. For this reason it may be found that the patient cooperates better in the occupational therapy department than in physiotherapy or in the ward, where there is perhaps more movement

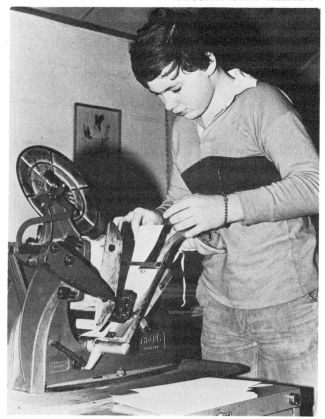

**Fig. 7.5**   Printing, which requires concentration and accuracy in putting the paper into position, provides a quick and satisfying end result for the impatient young person with head injury. He also gains practice in standing, balance and coordination.

going on all round him. Activities where the patient is sitting with a table in front of him helps him to feel secure. They may need to sit at a table by themselves where they can concentrate, or they may need to work with another carefully chosen patient who will set a good example. The patient may need to sit facing the rest of the room so that he can see what is making the noise: or he may be better facing away from distractions. After head injury, patients are frequently oversensitive to noise which can prove yet another distraction.

These feelings of insecurity can be made worse by poor memory which is often a problem after head injury. Patients may need repeated explanation of their programme or they may need constant repetition of what happened to them or where they are. During activity they need very careful and probably repeated explanation of what they are doing. The patient needs to be told the answers to his questions and then gradually he should be encouraged to produce the answers for himself.

Such memory retraining may need to be continued over a long period. Short-term memory defects may limit the patient's ability to follow verbal or written instruction so that it is necessary to use visual or auditory clues to help the patient to remember. Activities which interest the patient may help, as may repetition of an activity. Long-term memory defects may contribute to the patient's inability to perform the same tasks from day to day. It may mean that he is disorientated and unable to follow a simple routine. For these patients it is vitally important to keep the daily programme simple and not to change the routine. He should sit in the same place, be treated by the same therapist and probably be given repetitive tasks. Some patients feel it is cheating to use a notebook to remind themselves, but any method which might help should be resorted to and used constantly. Practical and familiar tasks may be easier for the patient and so will help to provide achievement.

Support and help in the earlier stages is most important if the patient is to overcome his insecurity and make progress. For this reason in many cases it may be helpful in the earlier stages for the patient to learn to relate to one therapist. Having found he can relate to one person he should then have confidence to relate to others. This 'weaning-off' must be done at the right time so that the patient does not become overdependent.

Success in activity is necessary if the patient is to progress. He must also learn to accept failure — but first he must find what he can do and build up some sense of security and confidence in himself. Sessions should be carefully planned from the beginning so that activities he finds more difficult are put in the early part of the session. Sessions should finish with a success.

With patients who have some insight it is hardly surprising that they may be depressed. Some, perhaps with less insight, may be euphoric. Both states may lead to poor concentration and a poor level of achievement. Activities should be carefully chosen so that a realistic standard can be set. It is easy for the therapist to accept normally unacceptable levels of achievement because of her understanding of the patient's situation. However, most patients know when they have or have not done their best and poor work should not be accepted: to do so would only reduce the patient's trust in the therapist.

Many patients with head injuries have little sense of responsibility. This often relates to their previous personality, social and work background. By expecting a reasonable standard of work and an acceptable level of behaviour, and by gradually encouraging him to take responsibility and use his initiative, the therapist should enable the patient to recover this aspect. Head-injured patients also often lack the ability to foresee the results of their actions so that they act impulsively. This may well be only an exaggeration of their previous personality (especially in the younger patients), but it is important to try to modify this behaviour as it may produce problems in employment.

It is difficult to produce any change in the level of achievement of a patient if he is not well motivated. If a patient does not have insight he may not be motivated because he cannot see the reason for the hard work involved in getting better: perhaps he cannot foresee the future, or reason through. If he has insight he may become so depressed it may have to be the therapist who provides the motivation — and this can only be achieved through her good relationship with the patient. Management of physical problems is usually relatively easy, and for the patient with no intellectual or perceptual deficit it is easy to give him relevant tasks. In practice, however, most rehabilitation units will not have patients with problems this simple referred to them, though sometimes a physical problem coexists with a perceptual one, but is still susceptible to conventional management.

## APRAXIA AND AGNOSIA

*Apraxia* is a term used when the patient has little or no loss of power or control over his limbs but he appears unable to carry out specific actions.

*Agnosia* is the sensory counterpart of apraxia. The senses are not impaired and the mental images are intact, but the patient cannot recognise what he is seeing, hearing or feeling, etc.

Although there are many similarities, and it is often difficult to differentiate between apraxia and agnosia, and perceptual difficulties, they are in fact different problems. Perceptual defects are concerned with the input side so that information going in cannot be sifted and sorted to the right places to be interpreted and acted upon. Apraxia and agnosia are concerned with the output side so that the patient cannot do what he knows he wants to do, or he cannot interpret the image he can see into something meaningful. The therapist must be sure the patient has no verbal receptive loss making an additional complication.

### Treatment of the problems of apraxia and agnosia

As in all areas of treating the problems of brain damage, it is best to try to concentrate on the more familiar and overlearned activities. A good deal of individual attention is required and, particularly in cases of agnosia, the same therapist should treat the patient.

If the patient has insight these problems can be exceedingly frustrating particularly in cases where the problem is very selective as with a dressing apraxia. To be hindered and unable to perform such a basic task, which prevents complete independence, can be exasperating and it may be difficult for the patient to understand the reasons for his problem. It can also be difficult for staff, not fully conversant with the problem, to understand the reasons, particularly when the patient is not consistent in his ability to perform. 'Is the patient lazy?' is a question which may be asked. Therefore, it is important to have made an accurate assessment with findings passed on to all concerned in treating the patient so that the patient is helped as much as possible to overcome his problems. All possible ways of transmitting information to the patient should be used in communicating and in performing activity with the patient — sensation, sight, sound. A verbal commentary may help these patients using the same words each time. The correct speed is important. Patients often try to rush in their desperation to do the task. Repetition of the task may reinforce his ability but must not depress the patient. Patients must be as happy as possible in order to get the best response, and to point out their disability too blatantly may be more than they can accept at that time.

## SPEECH AND COMMUNICATION
It is very important to work closely with the speech therapist so that the same approach is used and the occupational therapist can reinforce the work being done with the patient by the speech therapist.

Patients can often produce the necessary word if they are triggered: 'You write in your book with a . . .' This is not producing useful speech but it does help to give the patient confidence.

It is important to include these patients in group activities as they tend to be very isolated because of their inability to speak. Card games, such as 'sevens', can be very useful as it involves counting. Other simple card or board games provide the speechless patient with the opportunity to be temporarily in charge of the group when it is his turn to play which is what we all do normally while we are speaking.

Efforts to produce speech should be approached from every possible route. The patient should see the object, say the object, read it and write it, and feel it. In writing the patient is probably learning to write with his non-dominant hand so that it may be necessary to simply practise forming letters. It is always much easier to read a word than to produce a word, so that if a patient is to write a shopping list, she can perhaps do it if she has a long list, e.g. items from which to pick out those she wants. This may then enable her to go shopping if she can produce her list when she cannot find what she wants.

For some patients, the ability to read and write is of prime importance; but to many it is not, and some have never achieved the ability. Therefore, the therapist must not overemphasise this aspect if it is not appropriate.

In presenting all tasks the therapist should be aware of whether she is using just verbal directions or verbal direction plus demonstration. Direct commands with the articles involved in front of the patient can provide clues and help the patient to produce the words, i.e. 'Put the pencil on the book'. This will be much easier than asking a more abstract question, e.g. 'Where do you come from?'

To lose the ability to speak or produce words at will is a very frightening experience, so once the patient has been assessed all efforts should be made to work within the patient's abilities so that he is not threatened by his disability and his confidence can start to grow. If the patient is quite speechless it is very important that some method of communication is found so that the patient does not feel quite so inadequate and isolated. It is fairly unusual for an aphasic to be able to write more than the odd word when he is quite speechless and it is unusual for them to be able to draw or to use any other recognised method of communication: occasionally patients can spell out words on an alphabet board or point to pictures indicating they want a cup of tea, etc. (College of Speech Therapists.)

Where a patient cannot communicate it is important to find out how much he is able to reason and carry out activity without communication. For example: Can he match pictures? Can she put the necessary coins on the packet of sugar? Can she put the clock to the required time?

From this it can be seen that speech problems must be assessed together with perceptual problems. How much is receptive speech loss, how much is an inability to recognise the required objects, and how much is an inability to reason.

As far as possible, speech practice in the department should be about familiar things e.g. naming the ingredients when cooking. Overlearned words, such as small numbers in counting or money practice, days of the week and the months, can be used regularly and the success which is usually apparent in these instances provides some feeling of security.


## TYPES OF WORK WHICH CAN BE USED AS PRE-WORK EVALUATION

The occupational therapist may be able to have assessed the patient's adjusting to and learning to accept any residual disability such as:

Lack of self confidence
Fear of returning to normal life and to work
Communication difficulties if the patient still has some speech difficulties
Poor memory
Loss of noise tolerance
Poor concentration, which will be affected by his poor tolerance of noise and will affect his speed and accuracy
Lack of motivation
Loss of work habit

**Academic work**
It may be necessary to assess ability to return to normal schooling or further education. Patients who may need to go for training at a Government Training Centre or an Employment Rehabilitation Centre must be able to reach a prescribed level in English and mathematics so that it may be necessary to provide tuition and practice in these subjects.

**Clerical work**
This can cover a wide variety of jobs from the secretary to storekeepers who have to be able to keep simple records. This type of work can also provide invaluable training for people returning to the executive side of business where methodical, accurate work is necessary.

**Contract/assembly work in light workshops**
It is usually possible to obtain a variety of this type of work which can be helpful in building up concentration, work tolerance and speed while maintaining accuracy. Patients can be taught how to work in spite of their disability and how they can do the jobs with the aid of clamps, heavy weights or jigs. Is it necessary to change the work position or the height? This type of work can prepare patients for return to assembly line work or for sheltered workshops.

**Heavy workshops**
Patients returning to more practical jobs ranging from unskilled to skilled, can benefit from practice in the heavy workshops working with either wood or metal (Fig. 7.6). However, before allowing patients to work in these departments, they must be fully assessed elsewhere to ensure their safety in the workshops.


AIMS OF TREATMENT

The aims of treatment are: to increase joint movements, muscle strength and tone, including functional ability and coordination; to

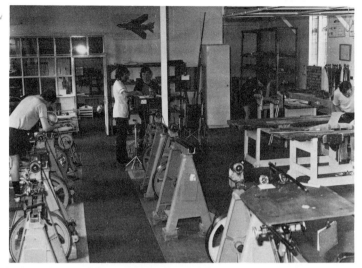

**Fig. 7.6**   Heavy workshops can be used in retraining as well as assessment.

increase stamina and work tolerance, and speed — if this is necessary;
to improve concentration, initiative, memory, self-confidence and
accuracy; to stimulate motivation and thought for the future; to
improve work habit, discipline of a work environment, acceptable
work standards and behaviour; to assess ability to learn and aptitude in
this area of possible employment.

It is important, particularly for men, to get back into a workshop
atmosphere after a long period in hospital care. For this reason it is
vital that there should be as realistic a series of tasks as possible and
that standard workshop practices are adhered to. Since in many cases
of severe head injury patients find it difficult to comprehend their
incapacities, putting them into heavy workshops may either confirm
them in their delusion that they are fit for work or they may have
enough insight to recognise their failure — which can be very
depressing.

It may be necessary to build up work sessions gradually so that time
spent in the workshops is increased to realistic proportions. At the
same time contact should be made with employers or the DRO so that
ideally the patient restarts work at the appropriate time.

It is useful to have facilities for:
   Bench work — measuring, cutting, filing of metal
   Use of various hand tools including drills, metal guillotine and
   bending
   Soldering and brazing
   Oxyacetylene/electric welding

Heavy machines, such as centre lathe and milling machine

Electronic equipment

Woodwork

Bench work — projects involving measuring and a variety of hand tools

Power tools — saws, drills, sanders, etc.

Wood-turning equipment, or the Oliver bicycle can be useful for physical exercise

With this type of equipment the patient can be assessed for:

Ability in relation to previous expertise

Aptitude with hand or power tools

Safety in handling tools

Speed and accuracy

When sufficient information has been gained, the aid of the Disablement Resettlement Officer (DRO) can be sought. He is called in by the doctor, who, using the information obtained, will fill in either a DP1 or the equivalent forms for those with psychiatric handicap or epilepsy.

The DRO will need some information, which will include:

Previous job — What is involved, is the job still open, is there a possibility of a change of occupation within the same firm?

Date of last employment — Did the patient work prior to the accident, did he have a good work record?

Patient's standard of education — Any previous qualifications? (This information may be useful as a comparison of his present abilities)

What are his principal work interests?

Is the patient willing to leave home or move house?

At this later stage the patient may still have many problems which he has to overcome — problems which are the result of the head injury or are the result of the long period away from work.

It may be possible for the patient to return to his former job. This is ideal, but obviously not always possible because of the degree of physical and/or intellectual impairment.

He can return to the same firm in a new and usually more menial capacity. This is less threatening since it is a familiar situation, but can be demoralising on the other hand. The patient is already known to the employer and the patient's previous work record may stand him in good stead, and his pension rights continue.

If a new job has to be sought, the DRO should be introduced as early as possible to assist the patient to find a suitable job, and he can arrange, if needed, further assessment of an Employment

Resettlement Centre. Training at a Skills Centre, Polytechnic, or specialised college for the handicapped, i.e. St Loyes.

Patients may be unemployable in open industry but be capable of sheltered work. They will need to be accurate, maintain reasonable speed and be able to work by themselves. They may have to transport themselves and they must be prepared to work a 30 hour week. Papworth Village Settlement and Enham Alamein are examples of such organisations, as also is Remploy.

It is also gratifying to note that after the careful assessment has been completed, some patients actually end up in better employment than at the time of injury, though this is admittedly unusual.

# 8

# Nursing care

## INTRODUCTION

The management of patients with severe brain damage presents particular problems for nursing staff, particularly if the unit also cares for other patients with severe and chronic handicap, such as multiple sclerosis or the sequelae of multiple severe injury. Some rehabilitation centres specialise in management of such problems but for the vast majority of cases the management of patients with chronic brain damage will only be a part of the nurses' duties. They often also have a feeling of slight resentment, frequently justified, in that they are the people who have to be responsible for the care of patients for 18 of the 24 hours of the day, and yet their expertise is rarely sought. It is not too difficult to find units where two extremes of this polarisation occur. On the one hand the collaboration between the nursing staff and the therapeutic departments may be virtually minimal with poor cooperation, no transfer of information and with many of the attitudes of either the nursing or the therapeutic staff contradicting the other in the day-to-day running of the wards and departments. At the other end of the spectrum, there are units where the nursing and therapeutic staff have made a specific effort to collaborate. An example of the latter approach was that at one unit it was decided that for all patients with brain damage or hemiplegia the method of treatment pioneered by Dr and Mrs Bobath should be adopted. In order to ensure a consistent approach throughout the unit, the physiotherapist who supported this scheme, and had promoted it, spent time both during the day and through the evening, and even came in at night in order to be sure that all members of staff who were handling patients did so in ways which were consistent. This was most effective in avoiding the irritations felt by the departments and therapists, or the nurses on the other hand, when a particular method of posturing would appear to be specifically discarded by another department. From the patients' and the relatives' point of view, it allowed a consistent approach to be made which could then be carried on at home as well.

Another problem which rapidly becomes apparent is that the assessments which are performed in physiotherapy or occupational therapy departments often appear to have little relationship to what the patient actually can do on the wards, and it is only by regular staff meetings that such discrepancies can be identified and hopefully corrected.

## AIMS

Since the care of patients is carried out in the ward areas for most hours of the day, the aim of the nursing staff is to teach the patient to become as independent as possible, so ensuring that the rehabilitation of the patient is a full-time activity. The nurses' work with patients will cover all aspects of personal care, toileting and management of behaviour problems and, as mentioned earlier, all the treatments that are started in physiotherapy and the other departments should be supported and continued in the wards. The relationships between the nursing staff of whatever grade and the patients must be informal though retain professional respect. Since the patient seems so much more of the nursing staff, particularly the junior nursing staff, he or she will frequently see the nurse as his friend and confidant and will rely upon her to support and comfort him when he finds the work in the departments difficult or stressful, and it is important that these difficulties and stresses are reported back sympathetically to the departments in order that, if necessary, the treatment can be changed or at least a satisfactory explanation of its aims can be given. The next aim is that the patient should be encouraged to be as independent as possible and the amount of assistance given by the nursing staff should be the minimum required in order to allow the basic activities of life to take place. It is better that the disadvantage of slowness should be accepted in allowing patients to make drinks for themselves or to dress or wash themselves, rather than that all these activities should either be done by, or fully assisted by, nursing staff at all times. Sometimes allowing patients to do these activities unaided involves a specific risk, but this may have to be accepted. This is partly in order to allow the staff to assess accurately ability and safety levels and partly to encourage the development of independence. It is most important to prevent patients becoming helpless and passive dependants.

## METHOD

Even though, in theory, certain activities are due to happen at set times in the ward, precise timing of routine treatments should not be considered the most important factors. So although meals and therapy sessions have specific times, and where possible they should be adhered to, enough flexibility must be retained to allow the patient sufficient time and space to carry out an activity and the nurse should never complete an activity for the patient just to keep to the correct schedule. However, she must also assess an activity, within realistic time limits. For example, if it takes a patient two hours to wash and dress himself in the early stages after admission to a rehabilitation centre, this may be practical and realistic, though irksome, but if it still takes two hours just before the patient is due for discharge, then this obviously is not practical and the patient will probably need help at home to complete this activity in a realistic time. However, if it has already been decided that the patient will not yet be fit for work on return home, then possibly two hours a day spent washing and dressing may not be as unrealistic as it first appears, so long as improvement can be seen.


## PROBLEMS

The following specific problems need to be dealt with by an integrated approach. These are feeding and drinking, dressing, washing and personal hygiene, the prevention or management of incontinence, the prevention and management of pressure sores, the anticipation of behavioural problems and the integration of the patient with society in general and his relatives in particular.


### Feeding and drinking

Many patients who are transferred from the acute hospital may have been fed by nasogastric tube, may still have the soreness of a tracheotomy site or may have had faciomaxillary surgery, all of which makes eating ordinary food difficult and time-consuming. In most acute hospitals the nursing staff are pressed for time and will usually have chosen to feed the patient rather than to watch him attempt it unsuccessfully and messily by himself. So normally on transfer into a rehabilitation centre most patients expect to be fed and given drinks by other people. It is a little brutal suddenly to withdraw this support, so that over a period of days or weeks independence should be encouraged at meal-times and as normal a diet as possible should be given. Those patients who have severe spasticity following brain damage are frequently fed sloppy or minced food on the basis that this is going to be easier for the patient to tolerate. Unfortunately it allows little stimulus towards developing a proper pattern of eating and it is probably better if, under correct supervision, a more normal diet is instituted as soon as possible, and chewing is encouraged. With the active assistance of the occupational therapist and speech therapist, the time for reintroduction of solid food can often be gauged accurately. If spasticity is a severe problem, then icing the tongue and lips can be useful on occasions.

## Dressing

In the management of dressing difficulties, the nursing staff will collaborate with the occupational therapists. In the examinations carried out by other departments, problems of perception, dyspraxia and inattention may have been discovered, so that somebody who has a dressing dyspraxia will be unable to tell the inside from the outside of a garment. They will be unable to appreciate that two legs will not fit down one trouser leg. These problems will almost invariably come to the attention of the nursing staff first, and without the awareness of the nursing staff that these perceptual problems may exist, it is easy to write off a patient as being uncooperative or difficult. Once the nursing staff have made an assessment as to whether the person is independent or not, then the next assessment should be done in collaboration with the therapists, who should come to the ward to do dressing practices with the patient and nurses. At the end of these assessments, the therapist should advise the best method to allow the patient to dress himself as much as possible: in what order the clothes should go on, how they should be laid out before he starts dressing, and what, if any, fastenings need to be altered. It is possible to replace buttons with pop fasteners and zips by 'Velcro' strips, and these alterations should be done quickly within the unit and to all the clothes that the patient is likely to wear. It may even be necessary to provide mnemonic aids, either by pictures or lists so that the correct sequence for dressing is always undertaken. Assistance may be required initially from the nursing staff but in many cases a surprising degree of independence can be obtained by encouraging the patient to do as much as possible for himself and, as mentioned earlier in the chapter, not feeling that time is of the essence but that what is being sought for is independence. It is crucial too that the same routine is adhered to whenever the dressing takes place and similarly with undressing as well. In practice the vast majority of patients are able to get dressed before breakfast but the system should be flexible enough and those who have problems in getting dressed should be able to have breakfast in their dressing gowns to allow plenty of time and space and privacy so that they may dress after breakfast and arrive at the departments later than the schedule allows.

**Washing and personal hygiene**

This is another aspect of independence where collaboration between the nursing staff, therapists and relatives is essential. It is remarkable how physically repellant some patients can become through lack of hygiene; it makes it very difficult to re-socialise the victim. In addition to providing aids for independence, the services of hairdresser, and chiropodist must be invoked if needed. Special attention may have to be given to oral hygiene; after a head injury teeth may have been damaged, so altering occlusion, false teeth lost, or badly fitting, and in patients with sensory inattention large gobbets of breakfast or lunch can be stored in the mouth unintentionally to emerge at the least appropriate moments!

**Continence**

*General*

Training the brain-damaged patient to be continent plays a vital part in rehabilitation since it is such a social snag. If a patient is incontinent of urine or faeces, then though it is sometimes due to the brain damage sustained at the time of the accident it is at other times simply because the patient is physically unable to get himself to the toilet and then transfer himself on to the toilet, or he is unable to communicate the need to the staff. If a patient has commmnication problems it is extremely important that the staff learn as quickly as possible how that person indicates that he wants to go to the toilet. This alone can sometimes cure the problem of apparent incontinence. This can be achieved by a word board or a signing system such as Makaton, or by the establishment of a regular routine. It has also to be recognised that incontinence can be used by patients as a weapon both against nursing staff as well as against therapists and relatives, in which situation the section on behaviour therapy is perhaps more relevant! Assuming, however, that the latter is not the case, then when a patient has been incontinent he should not be scolded — discretion and understanding must be shown at all times.

*Faecal*

With the problem of faecal incontinence, it is important to ensure that the patient has a bowel movement regularly. This can be achieved most easily by a good balanced diet consisting of plenty of fresh fruit and roughage. Raw bran mixed with milk and sugar can be eaten for breakfast, though if the patient cannot tolerate this then commercially prepared bran cereals can be given. If diet alone is not sufficient, a regular aperient can be used. This is usually administered in the evening, e.g. two to three Senokot tablets, 5–10ml, Dorbanex or Duphalac. The patient should be seated on the toilet morning and evening, and it should be explained to him that he is there to have his bowels open. After two to three weeks of trial and error this method usually proves to be successful and its success will be its own reward. Some of the less active patients cannot have their bowels open without the aid of suppositories, which should be given at regular intervals at a regular time. If possible, the patient should be taught as soon as possible to administer his own suppositories, so making him as independent as possible.

*Urinary*
Urinary incontinence in the male patient can sometimes be overcome by regular toileting. As far as possible a normal toilet is used rather than a urinal. If, because of the patient's physical disabilities it is necessary for him to use a urinal, it should be used in privacy. A toileting routine is commenced: initially the patient is taken to the toilet one to two hourly, and the interval is extended to two to three hourly. By this stage the patient is usually socially 'dry' and able to partially control his bladder. If he is improving physically, then going to the toilet is no longer such an enormous effort. Toilet interval during the day is then extended to three to four hourly, and four hourly at night, and all being well the patient is continuing to improve. It will have taken about six weeks to have reached this stage. When the patient has been 'dry' for several weeks on this routine, he is then toileted last thing at night and first thing in the morning (and throughout the day on demand). Careful observation and accurate records must be kept at this stage because if the patient is not continent by toileting on demand the routine must be reintroduced and toileting on demand can be tried again at a later stage of his rehabilitation. The same routine is carried out for the female patients. Bedpans, which the patient may have got used to during her stay in an acute ward, are rarely used. Commode chairs are used at night, partially because these can be coped with more easily at home if the procedure does not succeed eventually.

If it proves impossible to help the patient to overcome urinary incontinence, appliances and possibly catheterisation will be considered. The surgical fitter should be asked to call and advise on a suitable appliance. For the male patient the most popular and effective appliance is the Stoke Mandeville Condom Appliance, but this can only be used in the physically mature patient. A sheath which has a hole pierced in the end of it is attached to a length of drainage tubing and this in turn is attached to a 500 ml urinary collection bag which can be emptied by a small tap at the bottom. The sheath is stuck to the shaft of the penis by skin adhesive, and it is usually changed twice in 24 hours. The adhesive can be removed by warm soapy water. The patient is taught as quickly as possible how to manage the appliance himself and to empty the collection bag himself — again this gives him independence. In the young male patient and the elderly, the pubic pressure appliance is used. This is strapped to the patient and the penis fitted into a latex funnel which is attached to a drainage tube and so runs into a collection bag. With both appliances the drainage tube is arranged to run down the inside of his leg and the collecting bag is attached to the calf of his leg, and the clothing modified by a zip down the inside seam of his leg.

For the female patient who continues to be incontinent of urine, the use of an indwelling urinary catheter is often unavoidable. Before introducing a catheter it is important that time is spent explaining to the patient how a catheter works and the advantages of no longer being incontinent can be emphasised. It is important that the patient feels that the decision is as much hers as that of the nursing and medical staff. If it is unavoidable to catheterise her but she has been enjoying an active sexual relationship, it is essential that expert advice is sought for her to help with the problems that will arise. If there is no one on the unit who is competent to give this advice, an organisation called SPOD, who deal with sexual problems of the disabled, should be contacted to counsel both the patient and her partner. It is also important that long-term problems associated with catheterisation, i.e. recurrent infections, should be discussed with next of kin. The catheter can be attached to a short length of tubing and then to a urine collection bag, which the patient must learn to empty herself. She must also be taught to do daily catheter toilets — her personal hygiene being of utmost importance.

The sister in charge of the ward should contact the community nurse who will be caring for the patient after discharge and find out which bladder washout and catheter change routines she will be able to cope with on the district. It is unfair on both the community nurse and the patient to start elaborate routines in the ward that will be impossible to continue in the community.


### Pressure sores

These have a variety of synonyms (bed sores, lack of tissue viability) and may be present to either a minor or major degree. For those patients with areas at risk but with unbroken skin, it may be sufficient to ensure that the pressure on such areas is relieved by turning regularly. There is a vast range of beds and mattresses designed to reduce the risk of developing pressure sores, and for treating those that have occurred. They vary in cost from £50 to over £3000 each. Existing sores can sometimes be successfully healed by their use, together with good nursing care. In others, Debrisan seems to have a role, especially where infection is present, and there are occasions when skin grafts can be successful. But prevention is the best form of rehabilitation, so this is yet another area where right from the acute stage the long-term prospects should be considered.

## Behaviour problems

Behaviour is a difficult term to define, since to psychologists it means something considerably more precise than to the majority of personnel who have to look after patients who have suffered brain damage. In this chapter the term behaviour is used entirely in the conventional social context, since it is the most easily recognised aspect and one which frequently causes tremendous havoc for both the staff, the relatives and patients themselves, if it is disturbed.

Following brain injury the patient's whole personality may be changed. Some aspects of his behaviour, for example incontinence and aggression, may be a reversion back to childhood, yet the same patient at other times may be able to hold intelligent and informative conversations. Some patients may have very child-like behaviour and be grossly handicapped, but may still have the sexual drive of a normal adult, which may present big problems because of the associated disinhibition. It is also possible during the acute stages of treatment and through rehabilitation, that new behaviour patterns are learnt, though this will be referred to again later in the last chapter referring to behaviour modification.

It would be perfectly fair to mention that behaviour problems occur in any department or all departments but the reason that they are discussed more fully in this particular chapter is because the nursing staff will have to tolerate behaviour disorder for a great deal longer than any other department in the rehabilitation centre, so therefore their role in behaviour modification and control is crucial. It is also one more area where the need for good communication is essential since patients can easily learn to play one department off against another. Equally, it is possible for staff never to take the word of a patient as being true and so allow many misunderstandings to develop between departments which need not arise.

Probably the two most disturbing behaviour alterations are those of aggression and sexual disinhibition.

*Aggression*

This may be either physical or verbal, may be directed to staff, relatives or patients. On the whole, physical aggression is relatively rare, though threatening postures and behaviour patterns are often initiated. This is always a field for potential conflict since handling the aggressive patient requires an experience which is outside the normal training of the vast majority of staff who find themselves suddenly having to cope with it with little preparation. Probably the whole medical, paramedical and nursing profession as groups, could learn a lot from the language of body communication, as so ably depicted by Dr Desmond Morris, and so be able to interpret more of the wishes of people who have lost conventional communication through loss of language. In a rehabilitation centre the inability to communicate is one of the biggest handicaps for a patient and being unable to get what he wants by ordinary communication, shouts and obscenities and violence may follow. Usually the phase is transient, lasting only for a few days or a few weeks, but occasionally the patient may remain unpredictably violent, particularly towards his family, and this can be one of the causes of subsequent disruption of a family unit. The most important aspect of helping a patient towards an acceptable behaviour pattern is complete consistency between the staff in all departments. As soon as one department appreciates that there is a behaviour problem with one patient, all staff involved in the care and rehabilitation must discuss how to cope with him and how to react consistently to the behaviour pattern, and as soon as a plan of action has been established the relatives are involved actively with it. Usually the reward system is introduced which will either simply be praise or some material good, i.e. sweets or cigarettes, so that good behaviour is rewarded. Socially unacceptable behaviour has to be completely ignored though the interests also of staff and patients cannot be prejudiced.

*Incontinence*

For the vast majority of patients incontinence is an embarrassing and distasteful handicap, but for some patients it is possible to use it as one of the easiest ways of gaining attention or to opt out of therapy sessions which may be too difficult. These are the sort of patterns which can be learned very rapidly by a patient in the earlier stages of rehabilitation and altering this particular pattern can be time-consuming and difficult. Again, it has to be done on the reward system, either by tokens, small rewards such as cigarettes or sweets (however ethically dubious the cigarettes may be) and by making it plain without scolding that incontinence is socially unacceptable, and also wherever possible insisting that the patient clears up the mess that he has made. This approach does presuppose that it can be established that there is physical control present and that the other methods discussed earlier in the chapter are inappropriate for the control of incontinence in the patients with behaviour disorder.

*Altered sexuality*

Often one of the greatest problems for both male and female brain-damaged patients, especially those in the younger age group, is that of disinhibition. It is sometimes more obvious in male patients who can then be especially difficult in mixed company. The altered behaviour may range from the very mild backchat frequently experienced by nursing staff who care for patients in orthopaedic wards, to the more unacceptable and determined attempts to force the nursing staff to have some form of sexual intercourse with the patients or it may take the form of sexual encounters between patients, either of the same or the opposite sex. One of the other common behaviour problems which causes much distress for all concerned, is that of masturbation in public, since at this stage the patients feel no inhibition and may even thoroughly enjoy having an audience, especially if they react by either horror, disgust or amusement. Attempts to be intimate with any member of staff should be corrected firmly at the time, without fuss, and sufficient time taken to discuss the behaviour with the patient and its unacceptability explained to him or her. This is important whether or not anybody else is available for chaperoning at the time. There is usually little point in attempting to discuss the matter later, since by that time the incident is probably forgotten. Should a patient start to masturbate publicly, the best solution is that he or she should be taken to a separate room, again explaining the reasons for so doing. It is important to be reasonably optimistic about the problem since it is a phase through which many patients pass on the path towards recovery and provided the measures to correct it are not too draconian, may leave little subsequent trauma.

However, in the long term, problems of sexuality may still be a serious worry to patients or their relatives and this may either be because of increased or decreased sexuality, or because of a personality change when the partner who has been unaffected may feel physically or mentally repelled. In such circumstances, specialist advice should be sought where possible, and organisations do exist to provide this help. Not all members of nursing and therapeutic staff will feel competent or qualified to try and counsel, and if this is so then the most that they should attempt is not to appear shocked by the questions and actions of patients, but try to correct them reasonably and if they feel that it is beyond their competence to deal with, to ensure that the message is passed on and the problems are not suppressed to become bigger ones later. On units where a clinical psychologist is in a position to give good advice, their help here is also invaluable.


## REINTEGRATION INTO THE COMMUNITY

The nursing staff have a major role in helping the patient to get back into the family. This starts right from the very beginning in the acute stage and continues all the way through the rest of rehabilitation, since the nurses will see more of the relatives than any other single group of staff. They consequently need to be extremely well informed as to the activities that are taking place within the departments. In an ideal situation, during the daytime when the work load is relatively light, the nurses should be encouraged to participate in the work being undertaken in the therapeutic departments. They are then in a far better situation to answer questions by relatives and to help with the retraining both of the patient and those who are subsequently going to care for him.

During the stage of reintegration into the community many problems arise for nursing staff as to how much responsibility to leave with either the patients or the relatives. It is during this stage, when the patient is resentful of being constrained, that some of the biggest areas of friction can arise. Patients will want to know why they are not allowed to go out in the evenings to the local pub or to go to do their own shopping. In many cases the risks are only too obvious to the staff, i.e. the patient is unaware of traffic, but it is at this stage that, in consultation with the rest of the team, conscious risks may have to be taken and the support of relatives and friends enlisted so that the beginnings of independence can be supervised wherever possible. Errors of judgement will occur and some patients will be allowed off the premises who then either have an accident or get into an argument in a pub, and in many cases this risk simply has to be accepted in order that the majority of the patients on the unit can have some reasonable chance of returning to a normal life.

The question of the introduction back to the home environment is raised elsewhere in the book, but this is just to stress that in the early stages, although the ideal theory is obviously that the first contact with home should be at weekends, some serious consideration should be given to timing the first few attempts at return home to be done through the week in order that, if the situation fails, the back-up system is available. If, finally, the decision is taken that a patient will go home with his relatives for a weekend, it is very important that at the same time the relatives are given support and advice as to how to obtain readmission if the attempt is unsuccessful.

# 9

# Clinical psychology

## INTRODUCTION

The role of the clinical psychologist has changed considerably over the past few decades, from a diagnostician, involved in assessing patients on an objective standardised battery of tests, to a therapist, using objective assessments as part of an overall therapeutic process. This general trend is being reflected in the role of clinical psychologists working with head-injured patients. The assessment role is gradually being integrated as part of a longer term involvement in management of a patient throughout recovery from a head injury.

Although the assessment and treatment aspects of the clinical psychologist's role are becoming more integrated, for the sake of clarity they are considered separately below.

## PSYCHOLOGICAL ASSESSMENT

### Reasons for assessing the patient
The prime consideration in psychological assessment is why the patient is being assessed. This will affect the time that the patient is seen after head injury, the assessment procedures used, and the frequency with which the patient is reassessed. Consequently the several specific reasons for assessment need to be clearly stated.

### *Evaluation of residual intellectual deficit*
This may be present even though clinically there is no apparent deficit, such as the sequelae of a relatively mild head injury, or at a late stage in recovery. Even if a patient appears unimpaired intellectually and is physically capable of returning to work, it often proves useful to assess intellectual abilities to check. Concentration and delayed recall impairments may not be apparent on interview or in a home situation, but may present difficulty coping with work. Testing in this situation involves selection of procedures which are sensitive to mild deficits, rather than general measures of intellectual ability.

*Evaluation of specific intellectual deficits and abilities*
This will contribute to planning a rehabilitation programme, and supplement the assessments of the other therapists so that they can provide relevant treatment. In the later stages of rehabilitation knowledge of abilities or handicap may assist planning appropriate work possibilities. Assessments of this type involve a broad evaluation of a variety of intellectual abilities, though without detailed analysis of specific deficits.

*Relationship of performance to pre-morbid level*
The series at Chessington was unusual (see Chapter 5) and it is usually only possible to get an approximate estimate of a patient's pre-morbid level of functioning. This is based partly on educational and work history, and partly on the pattern of test results. In most instances some intellectual abilities are relatively well retained after head injury, e.g. vocabulary or picture completion subtests of the Weschler Adult Intelligence Scale (WAIS), and these may be used as a guideline to pre-morbid functioning. If a patient's abilities are commensurate with his pre-morbid level and it is physically possible, then work plans are likely to relate to his previous occupation. If, however, there is a significant discrepancy between pre-morbid level and present level of functioning, it may be necessary to consider alternative occupations. In this situation, one would ideally like to use assessments which have a known relation to work or activities of daily living. However, at present this information is rarely available and only broad generalisations may be made.

*Evaluation whether a patient is still improving or whether stable performance has been achieved*
The use of repeated assessments to determine recovery is a worthy aim, but difficult in practice. There are few measures with sufficient reliability and minimal practice effects that can be repeated often enough to provide an ongoing record of progress. If six months elapses between each assessment, the question of whether improvement is still occurring often cannot be answered at a time when management decisions are being made. Individual or small-group control subjects may be assessed to determine practice effects, but this is a time-consuming and often impractical procedure.

Serial testing may provide some information on the likelihood of further improvement. This is based on the assumption that if significant changes are observed between two consecutive assessments, then further change is likely, whereas if no change has occurred further improvement is unlikely. Again, the reliability of measures has to be taken into consideration. Prediction of long-term recovery of intellectual abilities is unlikely to be of sufficient accuracy to be of practical value at present. This is partly because the variables affecting those predictions, such as treatment effects, need first to be established.

*Evaluation whether the intellectual deficits observed clinically are functionally or organically based*

Psychiatrically based mental symptoms may follow a head injury, and psychological assessment may help to differentiate these from organically based symptoms. This is a particularly relevant question when compensation is pending, and the patient has no significant physical disabilities as a result of his head injury.

**Methods of assessment**

It is not intended to provide a comprehensive guide to assessments used with head-injured patients, but to indicate some of the procedures most widely used in clinical practice.

*General intellectual functioning*

The Wechsler adult intelligence scale (WAIS) is probably the most widely used measure of general intellectual functioning for the adult population. Its main advantage is that by assessing intellectual functioning on a variety of different tasks it provides an indication of relative abilities and deficits as well as an overall measure of intellectual level. Interpretation of WAIS profiles is largely based on clinical rather than statistical criteria and so the value of the assessment may depend on the clinical experience of the assessor. The initial stage in interpretation of a WAIS profile is the relation between the scores obtained and the patient's probable pre-morbid level. The level of the majority of subtest scores, or of particular subtest scores i.e. vocabulary and picture completion, or educational and occupational history, may be used to indicate probable pre-morbid level. If all subtests are below this level then generalised intellectual impairment has occurred, which is relatively uncommon. Scores on performance subtests are usually lower than verbal subtests. This does not necessarily mean that non-verbal abilities have been more markedly affected than verbal abilities. Tests involved in the performance IQ also involve speed of functioning and manual dexterity. Impairment of these may lower the performance IQ and yet not indicate difficulty in dealing with non-verbal material. The performance tasks may just be more intellectually complex in terms of the number of integrated intellectual abilities required for their completion.

If some subtest scores are significantly lower (i.e. by more than three age-scaled scores) than the overall level of scores, they may all involve a particular group of abilities. These abilities which may be impaired and indicated by patterns of subtest scores are shown in Table 9.1.

**Table 9.1** Table of psychological assessments

| Ability | WAIS | Other tests |
|---|---|---|
| a. General intellectual functioning | Full scale IQ | Raven's progressive matrices |
| b. Memory | Backward digit span | *Verbal* Wechsler logical memory, associate learning, Babcock sentence learning, Hebb digit supraspan *Visual* Benton visual retention, Recall Rey-Osterreith Kimura recurring figures |
| c. Visuospatial | Block design Object assembly | Cube counting Gollen incomplete figures Rey-Osterreith copying Warrington non-verbal retention |
| d. Language | Vocabulary Comprehension Similarities Information | Token test Object naming Fluency |
| e. Reasoning | Comprehension Similarities Picture arrangement | Modified card sorting test |
| f. Sequential | Picture arrangement Digit symbol | ? |
| g. Manual dexterity | $PIQ < VIQ$ Digit symbol Block design Picture arrangement Object assembly | Crawford small parts dexterity test |
| h. Concentration | ? | Cancellation tasks |

$P$ = performance, $V$ = verbal.

Many subtests are measuring several different abilities and so it will be necessary to follow up the WAIS with more specific tests of different abilities to clarify the results. The time that has elapsed since head injury when patients are assessed on the WAIS is likely to affect the pattern of test scores obtained. Mandleberg & Brooks (1975) serially tested 40 head-injured patients and compared them with 40 non-injured men. They found initially, i.e. six weeks after injury, that the verbal scale was less impaired than the performance scale and recovered to a level equivalent to the comparison group within a year, whereas impairment on the performance scale continued to recover over a period of three years. Therefore, at intervals of more than a year deficits are unlikely to be apparent on the verbal scale. The reassessments done by Mandleberg and Brooks were at six weeks, five months, 10 months, and three years after injury. Even with these intervals, improvement in scores occurred for the control subjects, which indicates that effects of practice cannot be ignored. The relation between WAIS scores and other activities has been looked at with stroke patients, but not as far as it is known with head-injured patients. The WAIS block design subtest was found by Oxbury (1975) to relate to independence in activities of daily living. Those patients obtaining an age scale score of 8 or less at three weeks after stroke were not independent in activities of daily living at three months. Further studies of this type need to be carried out with head-injured patients, but it seems at least likely that similar predictive indices will be obtained.

Shorter methods of assessing general intellectual functioning may be used. The notable one of these is Raven's progressive matrices, which is generally used in conjunction with the Mill Hill vocabulary. These methods have the advantages that they are short, easy to administer and may be given by a non-psychologist. However, the Mill Hill vocabulary scoring is less well standardised than the WAIS vocabulary, and the score only provides a broad grading of abilities. The progressive matrices has the advantage that it can be given to aphasics and non-English speakers, but like the Mill Hill vocabulary only provides a broad grading of intellectual capacity. The progressive matrices test is often considered as a measure of non-verbal intelligence, yet it is more highly correlated with full scale IQ rather than performance IQ. This could either be due to the lack of manual dexterity component in the matrices or the possible verbal mediation of the matrices. As this is not clear, it cannot necessarily be used as a substitute for assessing non-verbal abilities. Although the total length of time involved in using these two tests is less than the WAIS, many head-injured patients are better able to tolerate spending a short time on each of the 11 tasks of the WAIS than the more prolonged concentration needed for completing the matrices.

The assessment of general intellectual functioning will reveal serious intellectual deficits, but if no deficit is apparent on these tests it is not possible to conclude that there is no intellectual loss. Impairment of frontal lobe functions or memory impairment may be present and yet not be apparent in general intelligence tests. If there is no general intellectual deficit more specialised tests need to be administered before it can be concluded that no intellectual impairment has occurred. In some instances the general intelligence measures may provide a frame of reference for the interpretation of more specialised tests. Much more information on the predictive value of these particular tests may emerge with the full evaluation of the prospective data from Chessington.

*Memory*
Memory is the single most apparent intellectual deficit resulting from a head injury. It is frequently noted clinically that head-injured patients have difficulty with recall and in the more severe cases with recognition. Assessments on head-injured patients therefore need to include measures of memory functioning.

Memory assessments may be divided according to the nature of the material to be recalled, i.e. verbal or visual, and the length of time material is to be retained, i.e. immediate, short-term or delayed recall. Learning ability is closely associated with memory and so the two are often assessed in conjunction with each other.

Verbal immediate memory span is usually assessed on the digit span test combining scores of the forward and backward repetition of digits. However, only backward digit span was shown by Brooks (1976) to differentiate head-injured patients from non-brain-damaged controls. Recall of verbal material is often assessed on the logical memory subtest of the Wechsler memory scale. Two stories have to be recalled immediately after they have been told as an assessment of short-term recall and again after a half hour as an assessment of delayed recall (some examiners use longer delay intervals). Wechsler's paired associate learning task is the most commonly used verbal learning task and a delayed recall of the word pairs may be used to assess memory. These two subtests of the Wechsler memory scale were shown by Brooks (1976) to differentiate head-injured patients from controls. Poorer performance was related to longer post-traumatic amnesia and hence the severity of the injury. There was no difference in the performance of patients tested late post-injury compared with those tested early, which suggests that improvement may not occur.

However, since the study was carried out retrospectively and the decision when to test a patient depends partly on the severity of the injury, this finding may reflect referral policy rather than lack of recovery with time.

The non-verbal parallel to the digit span test of immediate memory is the Corsi blocks test. This involves immediate recall of sequences of blocks of wood, but is less generally used than the digit span. Short-term visual recall measures are less well-established than verbal measures. The Wechsler visual reproduction subtest has not proved to be sensitive to impairment of memory of head-injured patients (Brooks 1972, 1976). Clinically it is often found that while patients obtain average scores on the visual reproduction subtest their performance on the Benton visual retention test will be indicative of visual memory impairment. An additional advantage of this latter test is that the copying administration can be used to separate out the sensory motor component of the test from the visual memory component. Recall of the Rey-Osterreith figure after three-quarters of an hour delay is another test which involves visual memory and has been shown by Brooks (1972) to be performed significantly worse by head-injured than controls, though only at the 5 per cent level. Again, the inclusion of a copying stage in the tests enables distinction to be made between visuospatial and visual memory problems. One of the major problems with all these visual memory assessments is that they involve drawing ability and patients with motor coordination problems cannot be assessed. The use of a continuous recognition task such as the Kimura recurring figures can be used to circumvent the problem.

*Specific abilities*
In some instances, such as when devising treatment programmes, a more detailed knowledge of a patient's abilities or difficulties is required. Also, if results on the WAIS and memory testing are unclear, further testing may be necessary to clarify the nature of the problem. Low scores often occur on the performance scale of the WAIS which may be due to visuospatial impairment, poor manual dexterity or slowness. Testing of these specific aspects of functioning may be used to determine which deficit is present.

Tests sensitive to spatial problems, resulting from right hemisphere lesions, may be used to assess visuospatial abilities in the head-injured population. Although brain damage resulting from a head injury tends to be less well-localised than other lesions, visuospatial problems may occur (Smith 1974). Tests used with stroke patients, such as those used by Oxbury et al (1974) may be of value clinically but appropriate normative information is not available. If data on head-injured and normals were obtained, the cube counting, Gollen incomplete pictures and Warrington non-verbal retention would have the advantage of not requiring manual dexterity for their execution. Copying of the Rey-Osterreith figure has been used with younger patients and so the norms for this may be more applicable.

The appropriateness of normative data is also a problem for many language tests. The use of mixed aetiology groups to obtain norms usually involves a large proportion of elderly or post-stroke patients. Comparison of the head-injured with these may again not be appropriate.

The token test, either in its full version or as part of the multilingual aphasia assessment, is used as a measure of auditory comprehension. It is sensitive to mild deficits not apparent on other comprehension tests, such as the PICA and Eisenson examination for aphasia. However, the memory component in longer items may confound results if memory impairment is severe. The use of a second response is generally advisable with head-injury patients because of the likelihood of memory problems. On the expressive side, the Oldfield Wingfield object naming test and fluency tests are widely used, and some normative data are available. Reading and writing are generally included in standard aphasia batteries, and so are more often assessed in detail by the speech therapist. Deficits in frontal lobe functioning are often not revealed on assessments of general intellectual functioning. They may, however, be suggested by reasoning difficulties, poor abstract thought ability, giving concrete answers and perseveration. However, the basis for testing is that frontal lobe-affected patients are unable to use incoming signals from their environment to modify their own ongoing behaviour. Nelson (1976) developed a modified card sorting test which is particularly suitable for head-injured patients.

Sequencing problems may be apparent on the WAIS subtests — picture arrangement, digit symbol and arithmetic — but all involve other aspects of intellectual functioning besides sequencing. McFie (1976) suggested that difficulty ordering the cards on the picture arrangement subtest occurred with frontal lobe damage, and was a result of perseveration, as patients tended to retain the cards in the order given.

Manual dexterity tests are available but have been little used with head-injured patients. There is, however, a need for quantification of impairment of fine coordination and dexterity for which these tests might be appropriate.

Concentration fluctuations are noted by the clinician during psychological testing but rarely specifically assessed. Development of this area of assessment seems to be essential since it is widely reported as causing problems with the head injured patient's return to work.

Personality change is reported in association with head injury, often in connection with frontal lobe damage. However, there is little empirical evidence of these changes, as pre-morbid personality cannot be determined from present personality profiles. A behavioural analysis of current behaviour problems leading to the description of personality change may provide more information and give guidelines to treatment than personality assessment using standard personality tests. Oddy et al (1978) used a subjective symptom checklist to investigate personality changes and found a high proportion of patients with severe closed head injury reporting symptoms at six months after their injury. Comparison of this group with a group of limb-fractures patients without head injury supported the view that there are subjective complaints which commonly occur after head injury but less frequently after injuries to other parts of the body. However, these symptoms appeared to have relatively minor effects on ability to resume normal work and leisure activities.

## VALUE OF ASSESSMENT

The value of the assessment will partly depend on the question being asked. The question of how a patient is performing now in relation to his pre-morbid level or what abilities are affected, can for many patients be answered in general terms. If this involves language impairment or a memory or learning deficit in a physically able patient, a detailed analysis of the patient's deficits may be possible. However, in patients with concentration problems, frontal lobe damage or very severe physical disability the assessment will be more limited. Prediction of recovery and likelihood of benefit from treatment are questions which can be even less accurately answered. However, neuropsychological assessment is a developing field and so if questions are asked concerning intellectual deficits, they should provide impetus for the development of techniques to assess the deficits and their implications for daily living.

### Assessment of functional abilities

The principles of test construction used by psychologists to develop assessments of cognitive function are also applicable to the development of procedures to evaluate other therapeutic activities. Any assessment procedure needs to be standardised in administration, scorable, reliable over time and between assessors, and valid. Clinical psychologists have used their experience in test construction to devise assessment procedures for other rehabilitation disciplines.

One problem in applying research assessment scales in clinical practice is that the scores obtained are not clinically meaningful, so that, while the scales quantify patients' abilities, they are not sufficient in themselves as a description of a patient for clinical practice. Two recent studies on stroke patients have attempted to rectify this problem by using a Guttman scaling technique (Lincoln & Leadbitter 1979, Whiting & Lincoln 1980).

These studies showed that stroke patients recover in a predictable sequence of both motor abilities and activities of daily living. Assessment items are ordered hierarchically according to their relative difficulty. Patients are assessed on items in increasing order of difficulty and the assessments terminated after three consecutively failed items. This not only produces considerable savings in assessment time, but also yields a meaningful score. If items were not a Guttman scale, two patients obtaining the same score might be able to do different activities. For example, patient A might be able to do items 1, 3 and 5, whereas patient B might be able to do items 2, 4 and 5, yet both get a score of 3. Knowledge of the total score provides no information on what a patient can do, only how many of the items. However, as the items form a Guttman scale, all patients with the same score will be able to do the same items. For example, if patients A and B both score 3, they will both be able to do items 1, 2 and 3. The score of 3 will be sufficient to provide a description of a patient's abilities on that scale.

Whiting & Lincoln (1980) found that an activities of daily living scale obtained from 100 stroke patients was also appropriate for head injury patients. This provides an order of recovery of self-care and household activities, though further validation is needed. These results suggest that the approach may be appropriate for the assessment of recovery of head injury patients on a variety of scales and the recovery of motor function is at present being investigated.

## MANAGEMENT

### Management of behaviour disorders
Psychological treatment procedures have been used with head injury patients, but with little evaluation of their efficacy. The present account will outline an approach that has been found useful in the rehabilitation setting, but has not been evaluated or compared with alternative approaches.

*Behaviour problems*

Behaviour problems after head injury are commonly reported and ascribed to the brain damage that has occurred. This often results in their acceptance as unavoidable consequences of head injury, which will recover over time, but meanwhile have to be tolerated rather than treated. These behaviour problems take a variety of forms, such as aggressiveness, attention seeking, overdependence, lack of cooperation, inability to concentrate, lack of confidence and unrealistic expectations, all of which are often labelled as poor motivation. The effect is that therapists are unable to treat the patient and the whole rehabilitation process is disrupted.

Some behaviour problems may be a direct result of the brain damage which has occurred, but patients may also be able to learn acceptable alternatives to the problem behaviour. Thus, if aggression follows brain damage, a patient may be able to learn to verbalise in an appropriate manner the source of the aggression and then some control of the problem may be possible. Some behaviour problems may be learned in the acute stages following head injury and maintained by their consequences during the rehabilitation stage. Overdependency, attention-seeking behaviours and unrealistic expectations may be established during the acute stages, but only present severe problems during rehabilitation when they become inappropriate.

During the acute stage of severe head injury, patients are highly dependent on nursing staff. They may need to be fed, toileted, washed and dressed for a long time. During this time they acquire behaviours appropriate to this dependency. They learn to wait for a nurse to be present before attempting to do anything, instead of initiating activities themselves. They rely on medical and paramedical staff for all decisions about their future and are expected to consider only themselves and how they can 'get better'. Relatives will show sympathy and concern, and help the patient in as many ways as they can. Thus in the early stages the behaviour of staff and relatives alike reinforce dependence and compliance.

During rehabilitation a radical change in behaviour patterns is expected. The patients become responsible for initiating their own activities, attempting tasks on their own, making decisions and planning ahead. Most patients go through this transition without undue difficulty. Sometimes, if problems arise they may be as a result of staff and relatives not changing their behaviour towards the patient in a systematic and graded manner. One advantage of transferring patients to a rehabilitation ward is that the discriminative stimuli controlling behaviour will be changed and so facilitate change in behaviour patterns. The relatives will also need to be made aware of changes in behaviour that are expected. If a patient is struggling to dress himself and says to his wife that he cannot manage, she will help him with dressing and sympathise with him over the difficulty. He is grateful for this attention, which reinforces her giving him assistance. If this sequence is repeated over a long period of time the patient will become more likely to ask for assistance, and consequently less likely to learn to dress himself.

Some of these problems may be dealt with by the application of learning principles. The basic principles of behaviour change will be outlined, but for a fuller explanation several texts are available, e.g. Michael (1970), Berni & Fordyce (1973), Ince (1978).

*Behaviour modification principles*
Behaviours are determined by their consequences. If the consequences of a behaviour are favourable for that individual then that behaviour will be more likely to occur in future. If the consequences are unfavourable then the behaviour will be less likely to occur. In order to bring about behaviour change, the consequences of those behaviours need to be changed. If a behaviour needs to be increased in frequency then it should be followed by a consequence which is desirable for that individual, called a positive reinforcer. For example, praise alone may act as a positive reinforcer. Praising patients when they try to feed themselves may increase the likelihood that they will attempt to feed themselves in future. Many behaviours cannot be reinforced each time they occur because the patient is unable to perform the behaviour required. In this situation reinforcement of successive approximations to the required behaviour, i.e. shaping, is used. If a patient is unable to concentrate, he is initially reinforced for working at a task for a short time, e.g. two minutes, the amount required for reinforcement is then increased in small stages, e.g. a minute a day, up to the desired level. This gradual graded approach is needed in almost all behaviour changes in the rehabilitation situation because the physical limitations of behaviour change are often not known.

There are also various ways of decreasing the frequency of inappropriate behaviours. One way is to cease to reinforce behaviours which may have previously been reinforced. For example, temper tantrums which have previously received attention are ignored. At the same time reinforcement of incompatible behaviours will produce behaviour change. Giving attention at a time when the patient is behaving appropriately can be used at the same time as ignoring temper tantrums, so that the patient receives the same amount of attention but it is contingent on different behaviours.

These are the basic ideas behind behavioural management, but in order to apply the principles effectively further reading is recommended. These principles may be applied to both the general management of the patient and by setting up individual training programmes to deal with specific behaviour problems.

## General patient management

Attention and rest are two reinforcers widely used during rehabilitation. The timing of delivery of these may provide an effective means of eliminating some problem behaviours, or avoiding the development of others.

*Case example*

Mrs A lacked in confidence. She was able to walk in the physiotherapy department independently, but she constantly repeated that she was afraid and unable to manage. The therapist, following up the complaints of difficulty, walked with the patient and offered encouragement and thus reinforced complaint behaviour. When Mrs A walked without complaint, the therapist was able to leave her to practise on her own, removing reinforcement when Mrs A performed the desired behaviour.

In this situation the therapist's attention was contingent on reporting lack of confidence and therefore Mrs A was more likely to report difficulty and less likely to walk on her own. The alternative response for the therapist was to make no comment when Mrs A complained of difficulty, but to offer praise and encouragement when she attempted to walk without complaining.

In a situation where many patients are involved in different activities in proximity it tends to be those who are having difficulty and not working who receive therapist attention, while those who are working independently and well are ignored. Patients learn that the way to get attention is to fail or to not work. The therapist therefore needs to make her attention contingent on participating in the required activity. Given that patients having difficulty will need help, the way to train a patient not to fail is to give non-contingent attention, i.e. attention is received sometimes following success and sometimes following failure. If tasks can be graded in difficulty so that the likelihood of failure is decreased, this procedure will be more effective (i.e. realistic goal setting).

*Case example*

Mr B was reluctant to complete a series of exercises in physiotherapy. He complained that he was tired and so was told to have a rest, but this may act as a reinforcer and so make Mr B more likely to complain of tiredness in future.

Repetition meant than Mr B became able to do progressively less of each exercise. When rest was contingent on successful completion of an exercise, then performance improved. Mr B was given a series of exercises, each of which he had to repeat a set number of times. Initially the number of times required was well within his capabilities and rest was given after each completed exercise. The amount of activity required before a rest was given was gradually increased, so that improvement occurred. Careful grading of intensity and repetition of exercises means that rest follows success, rather than reports of tiredness. The same principle is used by the remedial gymnasts in class and individual work.

Rest and therapist attention are continually operating as reinforcers during rehabilitation. Careful consideration of the contingencies under which they are operating can increase the effectiveness of treatment and help motivate the patient towards recovery.

## Individual training programmes

It may be necessary to set up specific training programmes to deal with certain behaviour problems. Patients with very disruptive behaviours or those who are very poorly motivated, or for whom attention and rest are inadequate as reinforcers, may benefit from a more structured programme. These individual programmes are based on the same general principles but the behaviours to be changed are more precisely defined, gradation of progress more systematic and contingencies of reinforcement more carefully specified. Recording of behaviours is usually necessary so that progress can be monitored and the effectiveness of the procedure evaluated. Various stages are involved in the design and implementation of these programmes.

### Behaviour analysis

Initial systematic observation of current behaviour patterns serves three purposes. It provides a record of current reinforcement contingencies which are operating and may identify those contingencies which may need to be altered to bring about behaviour change. It provides an indication of potential reinforcers for that patient, for example, it may be possible to identify whether a therapist's attention is reinforcing for the patient. It also provides a baseline against which the effectiveness of the programme can be evaluated. This baseline needs to be recorded over sufficient period of time that variations in behaviour pattern can be noted, e.g. whether the problem behaviour occurs at a stable or increasing frequency.

### Target setting

Targets for each programme need to be defined in behavioural terms. What exactly should the patient do that is different from what he does now? Goals can be altered as the patient progresses, but at each stage of the programme they need to be clearly defined. Initial goals should be kept low so that they can be relatively easily achieved which will reinforce both patient and staff by providing a success experience. The next stage of the programme may then be aimed at goals more difficult to achieve. The programme used with Mr C provides an example of the use of target setting.

*Case example*
Mr C was a young man with a head injury who was uncooperative in physiotherapy. He refused to do any exercises, complaining that they were painful, he was too tired and that he was not improving so they would not help. Initial observation indicated that he was receiving therapist's attention contingent on complaints, and refusing to participate in treatment. His goal was to be able to walk and he felt he was making no progress. His memory was poor and so he was unable to recall whether his performance was better than the previous day, even if any improvement had occurred. Initial records of his exercises showed that he attempted three exercises within a half-hour. These were lifting himself on his hands five times, bridging five times and rolling twice. The rest of the time was spent sitting refusing to do activities. The programme devised was for a target to be set for each of the three exercises. This target was initially very low so that he was very likely to succeed. When he met the target, he was praised, his performance was recorded on a graph on the wall, and he was given a rest. Following this the target was set for the second exercise. When three exercises had been completed to target he was allowed to choose what he did for any remaining time. The graphs of his progress are shown in Figure 9.1.

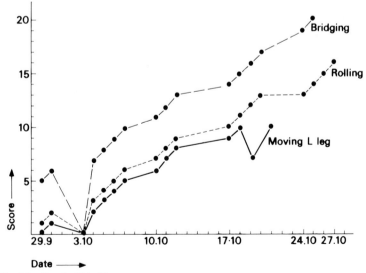

**Fig. 9.1**  Graph of Mr C's progress.

The use of graphs of this type have several advantages. Targets can be increased in very small steps frequently, so that improvement becomes more apparent and acts as a reinforcer. If targets are increased by one each day, rather than by five a week, the reinforcement, that improvement has occurred, immediately follows completion of an exercise. In the later stages of recovery after a head injury, progress tends to be slower and so not immediately apparent to the patient or staff. Records of progress serve to make very minimal changes evident to all and so are likely to act as reinforcers. This may be particularly important when the patient has memory problems, as he is even less likely to be aware of improvement without written feedback.

If graphs of progress are displayed on the wall, members of staff who are not working with the patient directly can give additional verbal reinforcement to the patient when improvement has occurred.

*Selection of reinforcers*

Three major reinforcers have already been mentioned. These are attention, rest and feedback of progress. During rehabilitation these are often very effective and may be sufficient to produce desired behaviour changes. However, when these are ineffective for a particular patient, material reinforcers may be used, e.g. cigarettes, sweets, weekend leave. The selection of reinforcers will depend on whether they can be controlled. Only activities or goods over which there is external control will provide effective reinforcement. If a patient can buy his own cigarettes, an extra cigarette will have little incentive value. Reinforcers should also be supplementary to usual activities and materials, rather than instead of them. Removing a previously freely available reinforcer is more likely to lead to lack of cooperation with the treatment programme than improvement in performance.

Reinforcers need to be given immediately following the behaviour which it is desired to increase. If there is a delay, the reinforcer will have most effect on the frequency of the behaviour immediately preceding its delivery. If a delay is unavoidable, such as when weekend leave, hydrotherapy, extra craftwork are being used as reinforcers, then tokens or points should be used to bridge the gap. Tokens or points should be given immediately following the required behaviour and then exchanged for material reinforcers at an appropriate time. These reinforcers, once given, should not be taken away, even when undesirable behaviours occur, as then reinforcing value will be decreased. The importance of tokens to bridge the delay between behaviour and reinforcement is especially important with head-injured patients who have memory problems. Establishing a full-scale token economy can be practical under some closed conditions.

*Generalisation*

Behaviour changes produced are under control of the environmental conditions in which they occurred. If a patient is able to walk in a physiotherapy department with a particular therapist, he will not be able to walk elsewhere or with his wife unless given practice in those situations. Similarly, if aggressive outbursts are controlled by ignoring them and reinforcing 'good' behaviour, this reinforcement needs to be carried out in as many situations and with as many people as possible, in order for the behaviour change to 'generalise'. When behaviours are being modified it is important that consistency is maintained by all staff, from the doctors to the cleaners, and by other patients who come into contact with the patient. Otherwise the patient will behave in one way towards one set of people and in another way towards others. If a behaviour problem has been modified by therapists, then it is necessary for the relatives and friends of the patient to be instructed in the behaviour modification procedures, so that the behaviour change may be maintained when discharge home takes place. When an individual programme is set up to deal with specific problems, it is necessary for the relatives to be instructed to carry it out or for the patient to be gradually weaned off the programme before returning home. This may be done by gradually decreasing the amount of time spent on the specific programme, while continuing to use general behavioural management principles. A gradual transition from material rewards and graphs of progress, to attention and rest as reinforcers, will facilitate this process.

**Evaluation**

The effectiveness of behavioural management procedures needs to be constantly reviewed and evaluated. For this purpose records of targets set and achieved, reinforcers given and generalisation of behaviour change need to be kept. If behaviour change has not occurred, it is necessary to consider whether the programme was correctly designed. There may be errors in identifying reinforcers, selecting targets and specifying contingencies. In addition the question arises as to whether the programme was carried out as intended. The possibilities are that behaviours to be ignored were not in fact ignored, there was lack of consistency among staff in their management of the patient, or that records were not accurately kept. These types of errors seem to contribute far more frequently to programme failure than the inability of the patient to change his way of behaving.

Comparison of behavioural training methods with control groups or alternative patient management procedures has not been carried out. At present time, behaviour modification is only just beginning to be used in the rehabilitation of head-injured patients, but it seems to be a potentially valuable technique. Control studies are essential before any conclusions can be drawn, though there are many attendant practical and ethical difficulties.

## Treatment of cognitive deficits

Cognitive deficits of head injury patients have been recorded and some have been shown to recover over time. However, there have been relatively few investigations of whether treatment can be used to enhance the recovery process.

Some investigations have shown that visual image mnemonic devices significantly improve the memory deficits of Korsakoff amnesics (Cermak 1975), individuals who have had left temporal lobectomies (Jones 1974) and brain-damaged patients of mostly cardiovascular aetiology (Lewinsohn et al 1977). Recent clinical work also suggests that these techniques may be appropriate for head injury patients (Glasgow et al 1977, Crovitz et al 1979). However, although these studies have demonstrated short-term gains in recall ability with training, the long-term effects have not been investigated and neither has the extent to which generalisation to other tasks occurs.

An alternative strategy to practising memory tasks is to train patients in alternative behavioural strategies. Patients with severe memory problems may be given calendar charts to tick off the days of the week and events within each day, such as meal times and therapy periods, as they occur. As a progression from this, they may be trained in the use of diaries, both to record daily events as they happen and to plan their weekly rehabilitation programme. Timetables and instruction charts may be used at home to circumvent some of the practical problems of poor recall ability. These methods do not serve to improve a patient's memory but they may enable him to function more independently in daily life. Evaluation of whether this in fact occurs has yet to be carried out.

The principle of behavioural strategy change has also been applied to deal with perceptual problems. Diller & Weinberg (1977) trained patients in head movements in order to compensate for the effects of left-sided inattention. Verbal cueing has been used to train patients to compensate for difficulties on Block Design, a visuospatial task (Ben-Yishay et al 1971).

## Future perspectives

Clinical psychology in the practical management of head-injured patients is a developing field and has considerable potential contribution to make. Refining of assessments may make prediction possible and enable more effective treatment to be developed. The control of behaviour problems may also help to increase the effectiveness of other treatment procedures. However, all treatment procedures need adequate control trials to evaluate their effectiveness using reliable and valid assessment techniques. This stage is now of paramount importance in order for rehabilitation procedures to progress from clinical intuition to a scientifically based treatment regime.

REFERENCES

Ben-Yishay Y, Diller I, Mandleberg I, Gordon W, Gerstman L 1971 Similarities and differences in block design performance between older normal and brain injured persons: a task analysis. Journal of Abnormal Psychology 78: 17-25

Berni R, Fordyce W 1973 Behaviour modification and the nursing process, C V Mosby, St Louis

Brooks D N 1972 Memory and head injury. Journal of Nervous and Mental Diseases 155: 350-355

Brooks D N 1976 Wechsler memory scale performance and its relationship to brain damage after severe closed head injury, Journal of Neurology, Neurosurgery and Psychiatry 39: 593-601

Cermak L S 1975 Imagery as an aid to retrieval for Korsakoff patients. Cortex 11: 163-169

Crovitz H F, Harvey M T, Horn R W 1979 Problems in the acquisition of imagery mnemonics: three brain damaged cases. Cortex 15: 225-234

Diller L A, Weinberg J 1977 Hemi-inattention in rehabilitation: the evolution of a rational remediation programme. Advances in Neurology 18, Raven Press, New York

Fordyce W E 1971 Psychological assessment and management. In: Krusen F H, Kottke & Ellwood (eds) Handbook of physical medicine and rehabilitation. Saunders, Philadelphia

Glasgow R E, Zeiss R A, Barrera M, Lewinsohn P M 1977 Case studies on remediating memory deficits in brain damaged individuals. Journal of Clinical Psychology 33: 1049-1054

Ince L P 1978 Behaviour modification in rehabilitation medicine. Thomas, Springfield, Illinois

Jones M K 1974 Imagery as a mnemonic aid after left temporal lobectomy: contrast between material specific and generalised memory disorders. Neuropsychologia 12: 21-30

Lewinsohn P M, Danaker B G, Kikel S 1977 Visual imagery as a mnemonic aid for brain injured persons. Journal of Consulting Clinical Psychology 45: 717-723

Lincoln N B, Leadbitter D 1979 Assessment of motor function in stroke patients. Physiotherapy 65: 48-51

McFie J 1976 Assessment of organic intellectual impairment. Academic Press, New York

Mandleberg I A, Brooks D N 1975 Cognitive recovery after severe head injury. 1: serial testing on the WAIS. Journal of Neurology, Neurosurgery and Psychiatry 38: 1121-1126

Michael J L 1970 Rehabilitation. In: Neuringer C W, Michael J L (eds) Behaviour modification in clinical psychology, Appleton Century Crofts, New York, Ch 4

Milner B 1969 Residual intellectual and memory deficits after severe head injury. Chapter 7 In: Walker A E, Caveness W, Critchley M (eds) The late effects of head injury, Thomas, Springfield, Illinois, Ch 7

Neff W S (ed) 1971 Rehabilitation psychology. American Psychological Association, Washington

Nelson H E 1976 A modified card sorting test sensitive to frontal lobe defects. Cortex 12: 313-324

Oddy M, Humphrey M, Uttley D 1978 Subjective impairment and social recovery after closed head injury. Journal of Neurology, Neurosurgery and Psychiatry 41: 611-616

Oxbury J M, Campbell D C, Oxbury S M 1974 Unilateral spatial neglect and impairment of spatial analysis and visual perception. Brain 97: 551-564

Oxbury J M 1975 Problems of research in speech therapy: a neurologist's view. Conference on Speech Therapy Research, London

Smith E 1974 Influence of site of impact on cognitive impairment persisting long after severe closed head injury. Journal of Neurology, Neurosurgery and Psychiatry 37: 719-726

Whiting S E, Lincoln N B 1980 Assessment of activities of daily living in stroke patients. British Journal of Occupational Therapy Feb: 44-46

# 10

# Remedial gymnastics

## INTRODUCTION

One of the original reasons which contributed to the initiation of rehabilitation centres within the services was the presence of a cadre of physical training instructors who, although they did not have medical expertise, had considerable experience in class work and the general promotion of fitness. During the early stages of the development of the services' rehabilitation centres in the war, these personnel, in conjunction with other disciplines, formed the backbone of the therapeutic input for the patients and in a similar way to that which the physiotherapy profession has developed from the original masseurs, so remedial gymnasts have developed from the physical training instructor of the services, and indeed many of the senior members of the profession now underwent their training in this way, though currently recruitment to the profession through the services forms only a proportion of new recruits. This built up the tradition within service rehabilitation centres that it would be the aim to try to make as complete a day as possible with a varied mixture of exercises, games, swimming, recreational runs and similar activities in order to try to stimulate the patient and exercise him appropriately at the same time.

Initially, of course, this concept was geared towards the rehabilitation of the physically injured, so as the patients become fitter and nearer the return to duty, parts of service procedures such as guard duty were included in the regime. However, when dealing with patients recovering from severe brain damage, this procedure has to be modified extensively, though there may be considerable merit in retaining close contact between the physically handicapped and those who have sustained brain damage, as often the groups interact constructively.

The tradition, therefore, of trying to occupy the patient's day as fully as possible led to the evolution of a class programme which changed every half hour and would then be followed by a relevant but different activity, and it was on this background that the programme for the rehabilitation of the brain-damaged was grafted.

As increasing specialisation of physiotherapists, occupational therapists, educational therapists, appeared, so the pattern changed but even at this date the vast majority of the patients at a service rehabilitation centre will spend more time with the remedial gymnasts than with the other therapists, except in the initial stages following severe brain damage. Nonetheless, even at this stage the remedial gymnast plays a crucial part. He or she provides a matrix of consistent and developing pattern of treatment for each patient which emphasises the fact that the majority of patients are still in the service. By concentrating on activities suitable for gymnasium and class work, unique opportunities are provided for the remedial gymnast to observe interaction between patients. Because of the close-knit organisation that such a unit allows, the work can be integrated carefully with the more specialised and one-to-one work undertaken in the physiotherapy, occupational therapy and other departments. It is also possible to study the role of active exercise and recreational therapy in the management of patients with severe brain damage.

## AIMS

Since such a large number of patients are seen together in the gymnasia the first aim is to provide an opportunity for evaluation of the social interaction of the patients concerned. Therapists in the gymnasium see almost all the patients each weekday except the small minority who are unable to cope with a full day's treatment programme or who at that stage have individual treatments only. They all arrive at 08.30 and 13.30 and each patient is expected to participate in the musical warm-up which takes place for the first half-hour of each half day. During this time the patient is expected to contribute as much or as little as he is able, be it in wheel-chair or otherwise' For the rest of the day both individual and group activities are undertaken in the gymnasium. During this stage the aim is to observe patients in smaller groups while they do both exercise and recreational periods and also when they are on diversional outings and visits.

At this stage, too, an attempt is made to reintroduce over-learned activities of service discipline which may well be familiar to most patients from before the head injury, though this is done in a sympathetic and gentle fashion. Nonetheless even at this stage attention to time-keeping, dress, and correct protocol are sought for. Most of all, the aim is to encourage interaction and development of social relationships within the peer group of the patient concerned.

ASSESSMENT

During assessment considerable regard is placed on the previous responsibilities expected of the patient. Some patients will have had supervisory or executive status, others will have had simpler duties. Wherever possible the handicapped person is given appropriate responsibilities within the group such as roll calls, or assisting other patients, right from the very beginning. They are also encouraged to take personal responsibility for their daily treatment programme. Other possible tasks are keeping scores during remedial games, and in taking messages between departments. As with other departments it was felt that the assessments are best taken over a period of several days to two to three weeks, and Figure 10.1 shows the type of assessment which was eventually developed by the remedial gymnasts and which formed part of the overall assessment of the patients. As will be seen, the tests are scored again on a 0 to 5 scale with the criteria for each score clearly defined.

**Method**

*The warm-up session*
As many patients as possible, irrespective of the severity of injury, attend this 30 minute musical warm-up period each morning. On arriving for the first session the patients are asked to attempt as much activity as they can, though obviously any contraindicated pattern will be explained to them. Instruction is by example, with the therapist usually situated centrally surrounded by patients rather than the more formal situation that the patient will have been used to. A variety of exercises is given, both in sitting, standing, kneeling and lying positions. Those who cannot walk remain in their wheelchairs or stay on a mat. The idea is that the session should be extremely informal and enjoyable and music to the tastes of the participants is used. At this stage, in addition to encouragement in the exercise the therapist will be looking for enthusiasm, motivation, attention and studying the patient's interaction with his peer group.

*Group therapy*
The majority of therapy carried out with brain-damaged patients is individual, but for this purpose group therapy is defined as any regime where there are two or more patients being treated simultaneously. There are a variety of exercises including walking and balance re-education, work for coordination, work on mats or benches which have been specifically designed to encourage patients to work in pairs. This method of treatment is very popular with most patients partly because

SOCIAL/GROUP ASSESSMENT

Note: a) The initial assessment must result from Therapist observation over a 7 day period.

| | Date | | | | | | Date | | | | | |
|---|---|---|---|---|---|---|---|---|---|---|---|---|
| | 0 | 1 | 2 | 3 | 4 | 5 | 0 | 1 | 2 | 3 | 4 | 5 |
| 1. Warm Ups | | | | | | | | | | | | |
| 2. Group Therapy | | | | | | | | | | | | |
| 3. Recreational Therapy | | | | | | | | | | | | |
| 4. Interaction with other Patients | | | | | | | | | | | | |
| 5. Willingness to help other Patients | | | | | | | | | | | | |
| 6. Willingness to accept responsibility | | | | | | | | | | | | |
| 7. Recreation - e.g. Trips, Visits, Shows | | | | | | | | | | | | |

Assessment Score

0 — Refuses to take part
1 — Participates when told — no enthusiasm
2 — Participates when told — variable enthusiasm
3 — Participates freely — little enthusiasm
4 — Participates freely — variable enthusiasm
5 — Participates eagerly and fully enjoys

| Narrative Report | Date | Date |
|---|---|---|
| Please comment as necessary on:- | | |
| 1. Behaviour | | |
| 2. Sociability | | |
| 3. Self Discipline | | |
| 4. Reaction to Staff | | |
| 5. Reaction *from* other Patients | | |
| 6. Punctuality | | |
| 7. Cleanliness | | |
| 8. Euphoria/Depression | | |
| 9. Depdendence/Independence | | |
| 10. Awareness | | |
| 11. Communication | | |
| 12. Swearing | | |
| 13. Continence | | |

Other Comments —

**Fig. 10.1**

it gives them the chance to use others as a measure against which they can compare their own performance and also because there is some element of competition. Many patients rise to these incentives and achieve a higher performance than if given the same routine individually. These exercises are also used when the remedial gymnast assesses initiative, response, and interaction. Many of the activities of recreation can also be used to complement the more formal approach of exercise and therapy. For most of the day the patient and staff are in a one-to-one relationship, so that any opportunity for a group to develop its own interactions should be taken. Even in a non-service environment a 'games afternoon' can prove a most useful addition to the regime.

Recreation covers a wide range of activities and the range will depend upon the ingenuity of the therapist concerned. For example, playing pontoon using different coloured counters or beads as stake money might be considered inappropriate during a rehabilitation period but it is one of the examples of games specifically used and can be seen to involve such things as manual dexterity with shuffling and dealing of cards and the handling of the tokens, spatial co-ordination, visual perception, communication, i.e. bidding and calling, and concentration and memory, together with other simple mathematics. Table tennis and other forms of games may similarly be used.

During this stage of treatment the staff will be particularly looking for the ability of the patient to communicate with a peer group, the establishment of relationships with new friends and any tendency to violence or aggression either towards the therapist or to colleagues. It is also particularly rewarding to see the tremendous assistance that a patient who has been at the unit for some time may give to another who is more handicapped than himself. This assistance may be given from another person with brain damage or it may for example be given by a patient whose disability is non-intellectual. This support from within the peer groups of the patient seems of prime importance. During the process of recovery it may often be apparent that increasing responsibility can be accepted by the patients and wherever possible this is encouraged.

Recreation off the unit is also specifically encouraged. (Wednesday is the sports afternoon at Chessington so this day is often used to arrange games, play readings, visits away to Wimbledon, the Royal Tournament, and to the many voluntary organisations such as the Lest We Forget association which are extremely active in this sort of programme. A similar programme was initiated on Friday afternoons at Rivermead Rehabilitation Centre where the therapists and nursing staff liaised on a circuit of activities including bowls, archery, dominoes and play-reading.) In addition to the value that the specific recreational activity might have for the patients, the opportunity to mix with and to see other members of staff and departments which were not normally in contact was of tremendous value. There was also considerable merit in members of the different departments of the staff meeting each other. This particular pattern of treatment has now been taken even further and will be discussed in the final chapter on possible methods of development which have arisen from this work.

**Problems**

Many of the problems experienced in other departments, such as incontinence, communication difficulty, the development of offensive language, and aggression, are just as evident during remedial gymnasts' sessions. Some of these traits have to be considered against what might have been acceptable in the environment from which the patients originally came. For example most senior non-commissioned officers and officers within the services are not so naive that offensive language cannot be dealt with, either by ignoring it, or by a summary and taut response which is frequently effective enough to silence the patient since he realises that it has no shock value in the environment in which he is using it. In fact most patients will tend to use the shock value of bad language in an environment where it has the greater impact, i.e. on the wards or in the therapeutic departments, since it is assumed (often wrongly) that the members of those departments are more easily shockable.

*Use of toys*

The Oxford Dictionary defines a toy as something meant for amusement rather than serious use, but during the process of rehabilitation following brain damage many 'toys' have in fact a relevant and significant part to play in the rehabilitation process. Most of the games and toys referred to were designed for children but many have the specific aim of combining learning with enjoyment (Fig. 10.2) so they are relevant to the retraining process following brain damage. Furthermore, most toys and games are graded for age and therefore

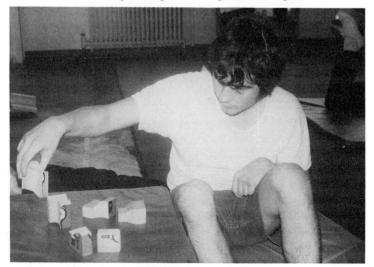

**Fig. 10.2**  A combination of learning and enjoyment.

allow progression of interest to be developed with increasing complexity as improvement takes place.

In the initial stages after head injury one of the most severe handicaps is loss of concentration which frustrates the patient as much as his attendants. During this stage games requiring short periods of mental awareness and concentration can be used to good effect. Simple games which require little memory for rules such as noughts and crosses, and card games can provide not only encouragement to basic memory but also by winning can give a reward for such concentration. As has been mentioned in another chapter, a game of darts (Fig. 10.3) can often produce feats of memory and calculation quite beyond the author. The example cited elsewhere was that of a patient who was totally unable to multiply two 19s and yet could do the subtraction involved in playing darts with speed and precision, simply because it was a thing that had been overlearned in his experience before the accident.

Another advantage of games is that they help to bring about at an early stage the element of competition and the development of an artificial and retrievable state of tension during the course of the game itself. Not only does this allow the therapist to observe the response but by discreetly allowing the patient to win on occasions, perhaps by bending the rules marginally, an enormous amount of reward and

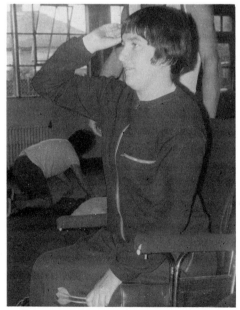

**Fig. 10.3**  Darts can be used for practice of calculation as well as coordination.

pleasure can be given for the feat of memory that this may have entailed. Furthermore, after a period of tension, be it naturally or artificially induced, the relaxation and satisfaction at the end of this can often be used to therapeutic advantage. Obviously the choice of game has got to be set at a realistic level and take into account the likely experience that the patient may have had prior to the accident.

Where there is a disorder of mood there is a requirement for an emotional outlet for the release of ordinary frustrations held in check so that the patient is able to 'let off steam'. This social interaction needs encouragement, for patients can easily withdraw into their own isolated world. During games and with the use of 'toys' there are opportunities for reassurance to boost the ego and to reinforce the feeling of belonging to a community (Fig. 10.4). Figure 10.4 shows the obvious pleasure that a patient is gaining from the relaxing influence of a game but from the therapist's point of view the patient's enjoyment is only part of the progress that he sees being made.

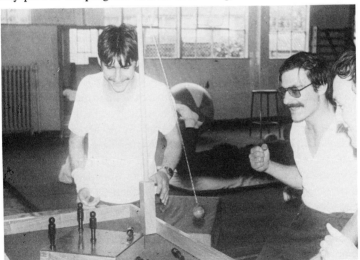

**Fig. 10.4**  Interaction needs encouragement.

Some of the material overlaps that which is being used in the physiotherapy and occupational therapy departments, which once more emphasises the need for extremely close liaison between every sector of the rehabilitation programme. Considerable care has to be taken to avoid an overlap that is unintentional and so meaningless to the patients. Some of the material will have wide application, for example, 'activity toys' can be for both non-walkers and for walkers. For the former, an excellent medium for treatment is an inflatable air mattress (Fig. 10.5). Patients who have minimal motor function are

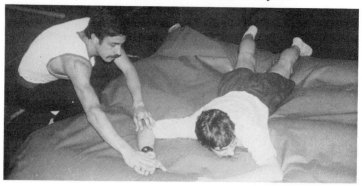

**Fig. 10.5**   An inflatable air mattress is an ideal medium for early treatment.

pleased with the response to movement that is fed back to them. From such simple beginnings movement patterns can begin to be retaught and encouraged through the patient's own curiosity and interest. For those patients who can walk the same mattress can provide an integral part of walking re-education since it specifically introduces the skills of balance and coordination and there is the advantage that confidence can be more easily re-established since a fall is going to be safe (Fig. 10.6). Thus it allows more adventurous movements and exercise to take place.

For those unable to walk, basic aids such as hand-propelled trolleys give increased mobility. Obviously those units which have a flexible workshop enjoy a huge advantage in this respect, but organisations such as REMAP (see Appendix) can often help in individual situations throughout the country.

There is a wide, but as yet unexplored scope for the new games, some electronic, on the market, some of which are worked through a television set. These games can be used, inter alia, to seek areas in which the brain-damaged can communicate more fully. One simple example of this may suffice. A patient who had suffered very severe brain damage and was incapable of holding a coherent conversation could readily understand the logic involved in the game of Mastermind and he rapidly became sufficiently proficient in this that he could defeat any member of staff, however hard they tried. The logic of the game was instantly apparent to the patient, and his economy of approach to it was incomprehensible to an observer but was devastatingly effective.

**Music**
In addition to the session allowed each day for warm-up, music can be employed as a background or for periods of relaxation. The setting up of small 'choirs' can be valuable as some patients with brain damage

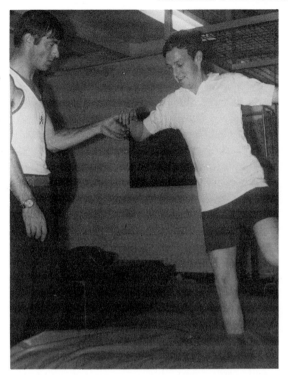

**Fig. 10.6** The same mattress can be used later for retaining balance and coordination.

can sing or play an instrument when more formal communication has been denied them.

In a rehabilitation centre with remedial gymnasts it may fall to their lot to organise a programme such as has been described in the early part of this chapter. In many units, remedial gymnasts will not be available and this task will fall on other members of other departments. But the integrating role is essential, and in order to provide a consistent approach some member of the team should have the specific responsibility either of coordinating the work of other departments or ensuring that there is a permanent matrix of therapy to which the patient can be referred when otherwise there would be a blank space in the programme. The evaluation of the effectiveness of rehabilitation is dealt with elsewhere, but if it is to have the slightest chance of success, then the approach throughout the unit has to be consistent. It matters less who has this responsibility than that it should be achieved.

Figure 10.7 shows that such an aim can, indeed, be achieved. In this photograph patients, therapists of all disciplines and nursing staff are working together in a combined treatment programme. In this system,

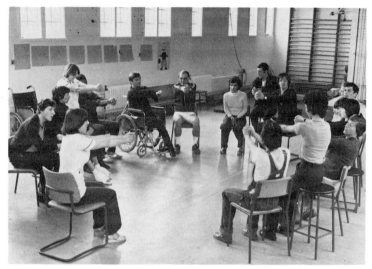

**Fig. 10.7**   Integrated classwork shows therapists, nursing staff and patients working together.

the background matrix of classwork is planned for each day of the week by a different member of the team, one day it being the remedial gymnast, another day the speech therapist, the third day the nurse and so forth. It allows for extremely close collaboration between the disciplines and seems a very potent development in the treatment of the severely handicapped.

# 11

# Social work department

## INTRODUCTION AND AIMS

The basic aim of the social worker is to work with both patient and relatives to plan the eventual return of the patient to the community. It involves assessing and offering support which relates to the emotional and practical consequences of handicap: this assessment and support may need to be offered to patients, relatives or to other caring staff. It will also involve offering practical assistance with accommodation, employment and training, finance and the mobilisation of community resources and services. It may also have to do with attitude changing.

In order that the role of the social worker shall be compatible with the other members of the rehabilitation team, it must be based on sound and established social work principles. For example, each patient must be given assistance and encouragement to make independent decisions and to take as much responsibility as possible for the planning of his or her future life, and it is important for other members of the team to respect this wish for independence.

The role that was undertaken by the social work departments in the two units that have formed the basis for this book, had much in common. At both units the task was modified by the fact that the social work department could remain somewhat aloof from the rest of the unit and so be regarded by the patient and relatives as 'neutral' territory. At Chessington the social worker was a civilian and as such not so directly subject to service discipline. At Rivermead the social work department was run by the local social services department and although situated within the grounds the line of accountability was not through the medical services at all. At neither unit were the social workers directly involved in treatment. Despite this, however, at both units the social work department participated fully during the occasions when decisions were being made and received full information from the medical and paramedical staff, and in return could frequently give much crucial information about the background from which the patient had come and whence he was likely to go.

Two specific problems arose regarding the work of social work departments within these units. One problem was the use of jargon, referred to elsewhere in the book, but which could sometimes serve to isolate one department from the rest of the unit. It will not escape the notice of social workers that those whom they might call clients have been referred to in this book as patients. This is not intended to reflect upon the use of the word 'client' since it is an appropriate one in some contexts, but for the sake of consistency within this book it has had to be sacrificed. The other problem which concerns all departments and the social work department particularly, is that of confidentiality. Obviously, medical, nursing, therapeutic and social work staff have as their prime aim the welfare and the well-being of patient and relatives, but when it comes to the transmission of information between departments, the issue of confidentiality can sometimes be difficult. The problem can be perceived either way. Sometimes the doctor and nursing staff feel that the social work department may have more information than they have given them at case conferences, and the social work department may feel they are being blinded by technology and that they have been isolated or relevant information withheld. It requires more than weekly case conferences to ensure that these attitudes are not sustained. Care, both in the selection of staff, and in communication within and without the unit are of prime importance. This issue of confidentiality is sensitive since it must be felt by the patient (or client) that they can place absolute trust in the therapist, nurse, doctor or social worker with whom they come into contact. Frequently, therefore, patients place a condition upon the giving of information in that it shall be given only to the person to whom they are currently speaking. If this information is thought by the listener to be crucial to the rehabilitation process as a whole, then the recipient of the information has a difficult decision to make as to how the interests of the patients may in the long term be served best. Sometimes the problem can be resolved by persuading the patient that they should themselves present the information to the other departments, thus overcoming the issues of confidentiality and transmission of vital information at the same time.

## ASSESSMENT OF NEED

### Information about patient (client)

Either before or on arrival of a newly admitted patient the social worker needs to gather relevant information about the patient and family. For many civilian patients contact should have been initiated by the former social work agency concerned with the patient, so that information concerning the patient's background, family and the nature of the support being offered, will be available. It is useful to formalise the arrangement so that a social work report is submitted from the previous agency as a patient is admitted. For servicemen, accurate information can be gathered about pre-morbid abilities and personality.

It is also helpful if relatives can be introduced to the social worker before the patient is admitted to the Unit. Because of the vast catchment area of the Joint Services Medical Rehabilitation Unit (JSMRU), and many other similar rehabilitation units, this is not always possible but it can be very reassuring for relatives who have been offered intensive social work support to know that in the next new environment a similar service will be provided. For civilian patients coming to Chessington and their relatives it can help to reduce some of the anxieties about coming into a service environment and can provide a useful link for relatives to meet other members of the team.

Through contact with the previous agency, and through interviews with patients and relatives, the social worker will gradually build up a picture of the patient's background, interests, accommodation and employment, and also how the relatives are coping and where support may be needed. This information will need to be transmitted to other members of the team, although as mentioned, the social worker will always be aware of the issue of confidentiality. Much of it will be useful to other members of the team, for example the former interests will be helpful to speech therapists in treatment sessions and the type and structure of the present accommodation will be useful to the occupational therapist.

From the information gathered the social worker will have some idea of how her/his role is to be formed in relation to each patient and relatives, although it may have to be modified throughout the rehabilitation period.

*Case example*
AB was a young serviceman who had suffered a severe head injury and whose physical and medical condition necessitated a great deal of physical care. The information that the mother had cancer but wanted to have the son home and to care for him with community support until she was no longer able to do so, meant that as the family would not be able to cope on a permanent basis long-term residential care would be required at some stage. Application for a suitable alternative placement was made early. This not only gave the family a much needed sense of security for the long-term care of the son, but also in alerting both social services of local authority and residential homes, it increased the possibility of securing a placement when it was needed at a later date.

## INFORMATION ABOUT RESOURCES

One of the greatest problems for handicapped persons, their families and indeed for professionals involved in the care of the handicapped is being aware of the range of help and facilities available both locally and nationally and through statutory and voluntary channels. All too often individuals and families struggle with problems for which there can be a solution and the social worker can be a key person in directing people to sources of information and help as well as assisting them to obtain it.

It would be impractical to attempt to provide a comprehensive account of the range of services and resources available, so the following gives only a brief indication of a few areas in which people often require practical assistance and information.

### Housing and accommodation

Discharge plans of a physically handicapped person will involve consideration of accommodation needs, which will be partly determined by the type of handicap and by the family and social situation. If adaptations and alterations to existing property are required (such as stair lifts, provision of ground-floor toilet/bathroom, ramps or other access features) application will need to be made to Social Services Departments who have a responsibility under the Chronically Sick and Disabled Act 1970 to initiate and carry out such works. This will involve recommendations from occupational therapists and often an architect, which will be based on an assessment of the individuals' needs and in the light of the existing facilities of the accommodation. If adaptations and alterations are not practically viable, it may be necessary to consider applying for council accommodation through the Local Authority Housing Department. Council accommodation can include specially designed mobility and wheelchair accommodation, adapted accommodation or sheltered accommodation. Some housing associations and voluntary organisations also provide similar types of accommodation for the physically handicapped.

If residential care is required, Social Services Departments have a duty under the National Assistance Act 1948 to provide this. Not all Social Services Departments run homes for the physically handicapped and may instead consider accepting financial responsibility for a placement in a voluntary home. If full nursing care is required Area Health Authorities may also provide residential care (i.e. young disabled units) or may consider accepting financial responsibility for suitable residential placements. The Area Community Physician should be able to provide information about this.

In the case of ex-service personnel, depending on the cause of injury or reason for having been invalided out of the services, the War Pensioners Department might sometimes accept financial responsibility for a residential placement.

## Aids and equipment

The provision of aids and equipment can come under the responsibility of various departments and because of the enormous range of aids available, handicapped people are recommended to seek professional advice when choosing aids to ensure that it is suited to their individual needs.

Aids to assist employment, such as remote control apparatus, adapted typewriters, page turners, can be provided by the Manpower Services Commission through the Disablement Resettlement Officer. Similarily aids to assist education are provided by the Local Education Authority.

Home nursing aids, such as ripple beds, mobile hoists, sheepskins, commodes or aids for incontinent patients, are provided by the Area Health Authority under the National Health Services Reorganisation Act 1973, through the District Nursing Services. Wheelchairs are supplied through the Artificial Limb and Appliance Centres (ALAC) by the Department of Health and Social Security. Family or hospital doctors can recommend a wheelchair and ALAC will offer advice, information and assessments for suitable wheelchairs for an individual.

Aids for daily living activities can be supplied by Social Services Departments, usually on the recommendation of an occupational therapist. The Disabled Living Foundation and other aid centres (see Appendix) can provide details on the type of aids available, how to obtain aids and will often have a display of aids and equipment.

## Transport and mobility

The availability of help with transport and travel for the physically handicapped driver or passenger can include: parking concessions for disabled and blind persons (orange badge, which is obtainable by application from Social Services). Information on rail, sea and air concessions for disabled people can be obtained direct from British Rail, or from the ferry and air authorities or from motoring organisations for the disabled (see Appendix) or from social services.

Information about the mobility allowance, a financial allowance for those with no or limited walking abilities is available from the Department of Health and Social Security, or from such organisations concerned with financial benefits and allowances, such as Disability

Alliance (see Appendix). Motability is a scheme set up to enable people in receipt of a mobility allowance to use it to rent a car. Details of the scheme are available from Motability (see Appendix). Motoring organisations, information centres and other statutory sources should be able to provide information on other aspects of transport and mobility, such as insurance, car licences, conversions and accessories for motor vehicles.

### Finance

The range of benefits and allowances can be quite bewildering. They can include sickness benefit, attendance allowance, war disablement pensions, and non-contributory invalidity pension. The Department of Health and Social Security provide information leaflets on each benefit and allowance but often the social worker will need to explain and interpret the contents. The Disability Alliance produce a Disability Rights Handbook which gives information on the benefits and allowances, how to apply for them, and how to appeal. Various voluntary organisations will consider applications for financial help in special circumstances and again the social worker needs to know where to seek such help, on behalf of the handicapped person or family.

This brief and incomplete indication of the areas in which practical help is often required demonstrates the necessity for social workers and others to keep up to date with changes in legislation and to build up an information bank on local and national resources. This is a daunting task, especially as there are considerable deficiences and variations in some aspects of provision throughout the country. Nevertheless it is imperative if the most appropriate discharge arrangements are to be made, which will enable the handicapped person and family to cope in the community.

Throughout the period of rehabilitation, the social worker can be involved in offering information and assistance in obtaining practical help, and, in addition, providing emotional support.

### COUNSELLING

The degree to which a patient can benefit from a counselling service will often depend on the amount of insight he or she has and the extent and location of the brain damage. This is because the patient's medical condition will often be such that any contribution will be difficult for the patient to make or comprehend. The social worker will need to have some regular contact with the patient to be able to relate to the difficulties experienced by relatives and by the patient, and to be aware of progress as it is being made. If the patient is able to benefit from counselling, it may be necessary at times to ask for the assistance of other therapists when there are specific problems. For example the help of a speech therapist when there are communication difficulties.

Wherever possible and realistic, the social worker should try to work directly with the client. In situations where this is impossible it is important to include the patient during discussions with relatives, especially when looking at future plans, even if no cogent contribution will be forthcoming. There will be situations when the patient is unable to come to, or effect, any decision, so plans have mostly to be made on his or her behalf, but this is a last resort.

When a patient is referred to another social work agency or when an admission to residential care has been arranged, a full social work report is supplied and all unconventional behavioural habits of the patient are accurately reported. It is difficult to find suitable residential placements for a head-injured patient, and a social worker should maintain regular contact with the home to ensure that both the patient and the staff are able to cope with the situation and that the needs of the patient are being met in the most suitable way.

One of the greatest assets that a social worker should have to offer is the time to sit and listen. By this the social worker can sometimes detect unexpected areas about which the individual is unsure or anxious. When this is related to medical or service problems, the social worker can coordinate meetings with the appropriate member of the team or service personnel to clarify the situation or to assist with the problem. Patients and relatives often express unrealistic expectations of recovery. Consultation with doctors can then be helpful to enable a more realistic outlook to be adopted, especially if both the doctor and social worker see relatives together after the initial assessment. This will enable the social worker to have direct knowledge of the medical information given to relatives and the opportunity of continuing the discussion to help relatives assimilate the information and clarify and resulting problems.

*Case example*
CD, the wife of a service patient, was a very practical and capable woman. The patient had sustained a severe head injury eight months before his admission to the unit and he had been unconscious for six months. On admission the patient had been assessed as having marked intellectual impairment, severe dysarthria and a left hemiplegia. The wife had been delighted that her husband had regained consciousness but had been hesitant to request any medical details about possible predictions for future progress. A gross communication problem shielded the wife from recognising the intellectual impairment so she had high expectations that he would be able to make a full and complete recovery. During a joint meeting with the doctor and social

worker, the wife was given a more realistic outline of the present medical situation and was informed that as a result of the accident and injuries, her husband would have to be invalided out of the service. She was extremely concerned about how this news would be received by her husband, and was worried that he would lose all motivation in his rehabilitation. Perhaps because of her own level of intelligence and because of the nature of the marital relationship, CD did not perceive the intellectual deficit to be a major issue or obstacle to having her husband at home. She worked closely with the therapists, and learned how to encourage her husband to accomplish daily living tasks while home at weekends. The tremendous practical abilities of the wife, her caring attitude and the fact that her own needs could be gratified by having her husband with her, offering companionship and security, enabled the patient to be accepted back within his family and encouraged to develop his remaining abilities despite all apparent obstacles.

The social worker involved with patients due to be invalided out of the services often has to commence with as much reassurance as possible that there is time available for resettlement procedure. In addition to coming to terms with a physical and mental handicap, the patient needs time to adjust to what often may be a dramatic change from a service orientated life to a civilian one. For many people, invaliding represents the loss of a stable job, financial security and close companionship with fellow servicemen. The resulting anxieties need to be explored and the individual given information about alternative possibilities and help in adjusting to the changes. The background and family situation needs to be clarified so that formal resettlement procedures can focus on future arrangements.

*Case example*
By the time Mr E was put forward for his resettlement interviews, the family background had already been established and a successful application for a hostel placement made. In looking at Mr E's social history it was revealed that his mother had remarried some years previously and that there were two children from this second marriage. The relationship between Mr E and his stepfather was strained and Mr E rejected any form of direct discipline.

Following Mr E's head injury and the family's expectation that they might be asked to provide a permanent home for him after his invaliding, they showed intolerance to former behaviour concerning drink and staying out late, stating that these problems had been exacerbated by the head injury. Mr E was independent with regards to all daily living tasks but was unable to organise himself to live independently without some form of supervision, and his attitude was often belligerent and slightly aggressive if things did not go his own way. Mr E was very reluctant to leave the services and desperately wished to retain a link if possible. The hostel placement in an organisation run for ex-servicemen provided that link and enabled the family to continue offering some support without having to accept full responsibility. The function of the resettlement interview was to arrange an employment rehabilitation centre placement in the area of the hostel and to take effect after admission to the hostel.

It will be seen that future plans are closely correlated to the attitudes of the family and the support that they are able to offer. Much of the social worker's time will be spent with relatives helping them to explore their attitudes and the personal implications resulting from the patient's head injury. This will involve working through feelings of grief, guilt, despair, anger, rejection and the implications on marital and family relationships. It is often by offering relatives some form of practical help that a social worker can find the means to offer emotional support.

*Case example*

The wife of a head-injured service patient was provided with service quarters near the unit (an arrangement sometimes available for service families) and sought the social worker's help in obtaining a nursery placement for the four-year-old child. During the process of obtaining this nursery placement, the wife raised the difficulties she was experiencing in trying to meet the needs of both the child and her husband, since she felt there was a conflict. It was also revealed that the wife had not wanted to have a child, so the decision had been at the husband's insistence. He had taken a major role in looking after the child so she now missed this support. The wife, in conjunction with the therapists, was able to organise her days in a structured manner, for example spending half a day with the husband and taking an active role in treatment sessions and the remainder of the day with the child. She was able to perceive progress being made by the patient, received information about his condition which enabled her to adopt a realistic attitude towards the future.

This case also stresses the need for the team approach both to patients and relatives in an understanding, sympathetic and informative manner in trying to help the family adjust to fundamental changes in relationships as a result of injury in order to promote an acceptable environment for both patient and family.

*Case examples*

When Mr F was admitted to the unit, his medical condition was summarised as 'severe intellectual and memory impairment' and also his physical abilities were extremely limited. The wife of this patient exhibited a great deal of anger both towards the service and also to her husband. The wife felt that because her husband had tended to put duty before his family he was partly responsible for his accident, and so had angry confrontations with him about this, and the implications for the family. His lack of insight and intellectual impairment meant that he had little or no comprehension of the meanings or reasons for the angry outbursts. The anger towards the service, whom the wife also regarded as partly responsible for the accident, tended to be manifested by a refusal to cooperate with various service matters concerning her husband, and by a hostile approach towards the service in general. She also tended to be defensive in her relationships with all the members of the team and this increased problems in the team relating positively to her. Mrs F initially used the social worker to express her feelings of anger towards the services and to raise problems that she saw in connection with the treatment of her husband. It was during one of these angry outbursts that the wife broke down and was able to cry. For the first time since the accident she was able to drop her defensive pose for a short while and express her own grief and feelings of loss. During this and subsequent discussions, it was revealed that the wife had been the scapegoat as a child for her parents' marital problems, and that her mother had been inconsistent with her affection towards the child. Mrs F had learnt to cope with that situation by withdrawing into herself and resisting making any relationships which might require a level of commitment which, if broken, could cause her pain. The radical changes within the marital relationship resulting from the injuries served to reinforce her earlier mistrust of forming a major commitment to any one person. Her own Catholic upbringing also resulted in a feeling of obligation and duty to remain with the husband. This attitude was not helped by her conviction that, had the situation been reversed, her husband would have opted out of any caring role. By helping Mrs F to explore her feelings of anger, grief and bitterness, she was gradually able to look realistically at the situation and see where and how she could have a constructive role.

In contrast, the wife of another head-injured patient, Mrs G, capitalised on the effects of the head injury to effect a positive change, as she saw it, in the marital relationship. Since the accident her husband had had difficulties in initiating any action and also had a short-term memory loss. The wife encouraged this dependency role, so that she could in future control his activities. For the first time in their marriage she knew where he was and what he was doing. She was unable, or unwilling, to acknowledge what she was doing, or the fact that it inhibited treatment. As a result she restricted in many ways the degree of integration that the patient could subsequently make in the community.

Part of the social worker's counselling role will be concerned with a patient's sexual identity and the attitudes of spouses towards sexuality and its lack. In couples where the head-injured partner exhibited confused, irrational behaviour, had suffered a memory problem or had some degree of mental or physical deficit, the able-bodied partner often had difficulties in relating sexually, even though during rehabilitation many of these 'symptoms' had been alleviated. With some patients and their partners, anxieties about the possible effects of sex on the medical state were a cause of anxiety, but for others previous marital and sexual problems had been exacerbated by the new handicaps and were now the central focus. These could sometimes be helped by factual information regarding effective contraception, aids, alternative positions.

Each team member had to be prepared for these questions to be put to them, be prepared to listen, and to have their own minds clear as to the extent to which they could give help or advice. This varied from therapist to therapist, but the most important aspect was for all the staff to know where to advise the patient to turn to for help, and not let the question simmer undiscussed.

*Case example*

A wife (Mrs H) who had performed a caring and supportive role and had encouraged her husband to achieve independence was completely unable to contemplate any form of sexual activity. The image of her husband during his confused and irrational period was in sharp contrast with the previous image of her husband when they had been able to enjoy sex together. She now felt unable to relate to him in this sense, but at the same time felt guilt at being unable to meet his manifest sexual needs. In view of the immense changes and readjustments in the relationship that had already taken place in a positive manner, it was important for the wife to feel able to resist the pressures of having a sexual relationship until she felt able to cope with, which in turn meant helping the partner to come to terms with the situation and looking at other alternative forms of sexuality, such as masturbation.

## Attitude changing

*Case example*

Mr J had been severely physically handicapped as a result of an injury to his brain stem. He had suffered no apparent intellectual impairment and was able to control bladder and bowel movements. By the end of his rehabilitation he had learnt how to feed himself, and had made some progress with his severe dysarthria and some degree of verbal and written commumication was possible. The social worker's involvement centred initially around the proposed marriage between Mr J and his girlfriend he had had for six years. There was a general feeling of concern throughout the unit that either the girl did not fully comprehend the amount of the long-term care that Mr J required or that she was marrying him out of a sense of duty. Discussions with them showed that they shared a very honest, warm and loving relationship. They were able to recognise the problem areas but felt that with support they would be able to cope. She felt that because Mr J had suffered no intellectual impairment and could still participate in decision making and take responsibilities, they could cope together with the physical handicaps. Her attitude and behaviour towards Mr J was as though he were an able-bodied person. During their weekends together they had formed a routine to cope with the physical care and attention that he needed. They had also experimented sexually and were able to enjoy a fully satisfying relationship. Both hoped that further progress would be achieved, but related all plans to Mr J's present handicaps and so were very realistic in this respect. By the time that Mr J was discharged from the unit a ground floor council flat had been provided and the necessary adaptations carried out. A day centre placement for twice a week had been arranged, as had outpatient physiotherapy and speech therapy. Contact had been made with the local authority social worker and a joint visit made to introduce the new social worker. Various leisure opportunities had also been explored and initiated, and it is gratifying to record that at the time of writing this chapter, the first child is due.

It can be difficult for outsiders to envisage why an able bodied person should marry someone who is severely handicapped. This attitude can reflect not only an acknowledgement that one could not react similarly; but perhaps also, underlying a professional and clinical attitude, there is some conflict in regarding this form of liaison between the handicapped and the able bodied. It would be interesting to know more about why such marriages take place, the personalities and needs of the partners and the form that the relationship takes over a number of years, and also to explore the difficulties that caring staff have in viewing objectively the sexuality of the handicapped.

It has already been emphasised elsewhere that flexibility is an essential part of caring for patients with severe brain damage. This flexibility is particularly needed because of the uncertainty in making accurate prognoses, and it is this same difficulty in giving accurate information to patients and their relatives that can sometimes be a source of frustration to all concerned. It is imperative that all members of the team, including the social worker, are aware that despite all precautions and care taken in making assessments, patterns of recovery will vary tremendously.

*Case example*
Mr K was involved in an aircraft accident and rendered unconscious for several weeks, and sustained other severe injuries. It was felt by the admitting hospital that he had no chance of survival and his wife was so informed. However, the patient did not die, though by the time consciousness was recovered months later he had developed severe flexion contractures of knees, hips and elbows, and furthermore the fractures which he had sustained at the time of the head injury were maluniting in a poor position. At this stage, his wife was informed that he would never be able to walk, talk or go home. A year after the initial accident, the patient was admitted to a rehabilitation centre and over the next three years continued to make progress to the point finally of being able to talk coherently. He then required operations on his eyes, his fractures and for the relief of contractures, and his wife was told that the patient might eventually be fit to go home.

During the four years of rehabilitation many discharge plans were initiated and discarded. They all related to the degree of progress made by patient, the amount of support that the wife felt able to offer and the expectations of the rehabilitation team. Plans initiated ranged from applications for residential care, hostel placement, placement within a 'village community' to accommodate patient and family, to the patient returning home and attending a sheltered workshop. The final outcome was that a successful application was made to a training college for the disabled to take a business studies course. This followed an ERC assessment. On completion of this course, Mr K was to return home and take up open employment with a sympathetic employer. At no stage had this level of independence been predicted.

In terms of the patient, the process of rehabilitation enabled him to be reintegrated into the community, in that he could take up employment, have an income and remain with his family. From the wife's point of view the success of the process seems a little less certain. Her husband has an impaired personality, their relationship has changed dramatically over the last three years and seems unlikely to regain its original depth and emotional content. She has also had to cope with severe temper tantrums that her husband displays (usually at home!) If open employment proves practical, the local Social Services Department (probably overworked) may not feel it necessary to continue offering support in a seemingly stable situation. The wife fears that she will be left to cope with the problems that will arise as a result of his survival and the rehabilitation of her husband, and she suspects that support will only be forthcoming if and when a crisis arises.

This sort of history is frequently seen, and demonstrates not only the need of flexibility in planning, but that stress can remain in the family long after the process of rehabilitation has been theoretically completed. Referrals to area social services need to be comprehensive and indicate the form of help that may be pertinent to the family. This may make it more likely that appropriate support is provided within the community, and also that families are clear about where to seek help, before rather than after a crisis emerges.

# 12

# Future developments

This far this book has dealt with the practical management of those who have survived head injury and who have sustained some degree of brain damage. It has been stressed in many chapters that a big problem is to separate out recovery that takes place through nature, from that which is encouraged by art and science. Every rehabilitation unit and hospital has its own apocrypha in which case histories of dramatic and unexpected recoveries occur, for which no good reason can be advanced. There is general agreement that nerve cells, once destroyed, do not recover, but there are enough patients who defeat this prediction and continue to recover over months and years; though until recently there has been no hard evidence to suggest how this recovery may take place. Support for the intuitive feeling that recovery does take place over many years is now beginning to come from the work of the neurophysiologists who are concerned with the recircuiting and plasticity of the central nervous system. Those readers who wish to explore this extremely exciting field further should read the works of Professor Bach-y-Rita (1980, 1981). A moving insight into the recovery following stroke was also given by Professor Brodal who has described his own recovery from a stroke (1973). While there is obviously some difference in the consequences of the brain damage after stroke, as opposed to head injury, many of the points that Professor Brodal makes in his paper are reiterated by people who have recovered from severe brain damage.

## OUTCOME MEASURES

If the effects of brain damage are to be scientifically recorded for the future, then not only do the severity of the original injury and the extent of physical and mental handicap have to be carefully defined and assessed, but also the quality of recovery has to be linked to outcome measures which themselves are repeatable and related to real life. Without such standardisation it becomes impossible to compare groups of patients studied in different centres or in different countries.

**Table 12.1**

| Classification | Outcome categories |
|---|---|
| Carlsson et al | Persisting coma; persisting dementia; mental restitution |
| Pazzaglia et al | Prolonged coma; partially re-integrated; recovered |
| Heiskanen and Sipponen | Permanent invalid; recovery |
| Vigoroux et al | Serious sequelae; nil/slight sequelae |
| Overgaard et al | Apallic; severe deficit; good recovery |
| Vapalahti and Troupp | Vegetative existence; recovery |

After Jennett & Bond (1975).

Professor Jennett and Professor Bond have emphasised this point in their studies of severe brain damage and have prepared a table (Table 12.1) showing the outcome categories used throughout the Continent over the last 10 or 15 years (Jennett & Bond 1975). It will be seen how ill-defined the outcome from severe brain damage has been. In an attempt to refine this, they have subsequently devised their own scale (Jennett & Bond 1975), but even on this the bands of outcome are extremely broad (Table 12.2). Current research is being undertaken into a much broader spectrum of outcome whereby, it is hoped the social and financial impact of handicap can be measured more precisely, and once this has been effectively done, then solving the problems surrounding the evaluation of rehabilitation can start.

As an example of early steps towards defining outcome of brain damage, significant progress has recently been made by measuring handicap of patients rather than simply giving medical diagnoses. The first work along this path was begun by a group working at Bedford College in London who produced definitions of impairment, disability and handicap (Table 12.3). These measurements were later used by Dr Amelia Harris in her assessment of the needs of the handicapped. The question of identifying handicap within the community was taken still further by Dr Agerholm in her study (1978). Finally, during the second stage of the Chessington research, the outcome measures assessed not only physical and mental handicap, but accommodation, employability, financial status, the amount and cost of aids provided and the level of dependency. Work is now in process correlating these

**Table 12.2**  Glasgow outcome scale

| | |
|---|---|
| Dead | |
| Persistent vegetative state | { Sleep/wake<br>{ Non-sentient |
| Severely disabled | Conscious but dependent |
| Moderately disabled | Independent but disabled |
| Good recovery | May have mild residual disability |

After Jennett & Bond (1975).

**Table 12.3**    Definitions of impairment, disability and handicap

*Impairment*
A health impairment is any loss or abnormality of psychological, physiological, or anatomical structure or function. It thus represents any disturbance of or interference with the normal structure and functioning of the body and the person

Impairment is characterised by a permanent or transitory psychological, physiological or anatomical loss or abnormality. It includes such defects as a missing or defective limb, organ, tissue, or other structure of the body, or an abnormality of a functional system or mechanism of the body, including the systems of mental function

*Disability*
A disability is any restriction or lack of the ability to perform an activity in the manner or within the range considered normal for a human being. In the context of health experience it thus represents any loss or reduction in the functional performance of the body or the person that is consequent upon impairment

*Handicap*
A handicap is an impairment or a disability that constitutes a disadvantage for a given individual in that it limits or prevents the fulfilment of a role that is normal (depending on age, sex and social and cultural factors) for that individual

measures with the severity of the original injury and the assessments done by the therapists in the early stages of rehabilitation, and it may be that different patterns of care will develop from this. Some of the early information is entirely predictable, for example, the longer a period of unconsciousness, the longer is likely to be the duration of PTA and the more dependent the person is likely to be. But a wealth of further information is awaiting analysis. Early results from the series suggest that neither the level of physical handicap, nor the associated injuries, play a major part in predicting or causing future social handicap, but that the inability to retain information or acquire new information and the inability to sequence ideas is of tremendous significance. This might suggest a totally new approach to the rehabilitation of brain-damaged patients, with less emphasis being placed on treating the physical handicap and a far greater stress on the retraining of memory and sequencing. For those who have lost speech and communication, there are other developments in store, some of them using sophisticated techniques, including communicators, which are expensive but may be of value to some. Other aids such as the Makaton signing system are inexpensive and yet provide a bridge for many; not only to give them a practical form of communication, but at the same time to be able to reinforce their powers of speech. The use of teaching aids and teaching machines as outlined in the chapter on the education department is also an exciting development, for here is a method by which programmes can be individually written and their speed tailored to match the competence of the person who is relearning a skill or a language.

## REHABILITATION RESEARCH

One of the biggest problems is the measurement of the effectiveness of rehabilitation. In addition to standardising outcome measures and the extent of the original handicap, it is essential to be able to chart recovery accurately and to be able to produce series where matched groups of patients are subjected to different regimes. This has been referred to throughout the book, but no wholly satisfactory technique has yet been put forward. For many drugs, a double-blind control is practical and effective and produces an answer, though even this is fraught with hazard, for if one drug is really felt to be significantly better than a placebo, the unethical implications of knowingly withholding drugs from 50 per cent of the patients being studied are difficult to justify. If it is difficult for such drug trials to take place with effective control, it is even more so when a physical treatment is involved because there are very few ways in which a physical treatment can be given and specifically made to be ineffective, for either the patient will be acutely aware of this, or the therapist who is giving it. It may just be feasible to establish, for example, whether short-wave diathermy or ultrasonics will be effective in relieving the pain of a muscle sprain, and by using untuned variants of the same technique, unbeknown either to the patient or the therapist, see whether in fact there is a difference between the two. This may prove a point, but it is of no use comparing techniques such as Bobath with Rood or Brunnstrom or other forms of physical treatment since it is not possible to make blind controlled trials. Other methods will therefore have to be devised for evaluation of the effectiveness of different regimes.

Two such alternative approaches to rehabilitation research must be briefly discussed. Referring back to the summary charts in Chapter 1, it will be seen that precise information can be obtained regarding the presence or absence of a specific ability. This has been taken further by producing more frequent serial analysis of those aspects of the physiotherapist's examination that dealt with locomotor ability. Figures 12.1, 12.2 and 12.3 isolate this locomotor score and show the abilities recovered by one patient over a period of five years. It was then decided on an experimental basis to record the locomotor score at weekly intervals and from this construct a recovery curve (Fig. 12.4). Visually this appears to be the sort of curve to which could be attached a mathematical function, and it would suggest that noting the first few points on the graph would enable a prediction for the individual to be made at a relatively early stage of recovery. The inherent error in this assumption is that the steps in the score are uniform, and this of course

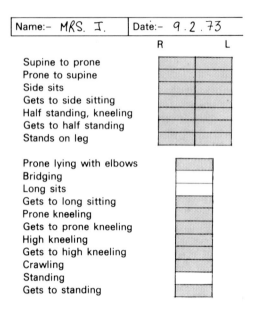

Name:- M*R*S. I.    Date:- 9.2.73

| | R | L |
|---|---|---|
| Supine to prone | | |
| Prone to supine | | |
| Side sits | | |
| Gets to side sitting | | |
| Half standing, kneeling | | |
| Gets to half standing | | |
| Stands on leg | | |

Prone lying with elbows
Bridging
Long sits
Gets to long sitting
Prone kneeling
Gets to prone kneeling
High kneeling
Gets to high kneeling
Crawling
Standing
Gets to standing

**Fig. 12.1**

Name:- M*R*S. I.    Date:- 10.5.73

| | R | L |
|---|---|---|
| Supine to prone | | |
| Prone to supine | | |
| Side sits | | |
| Gets to side sitting | | |
| Half standing, kneeling | | |
| Gets to half standing | | |
| Stands on leg | | |

Prone lying with elbows
Bridging
Long sits
Gets to long sitting
Prone kneeling
Gets to prone kneeling
High kneeling
Gets to high kneeling
Crawling
Standing
Gets to standing

**Fig. 12.2**

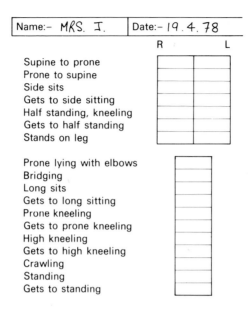

Fig. 12.3

**Figs. 12.1, 12.2 & 12.3** Three examples of locomotor scoring.

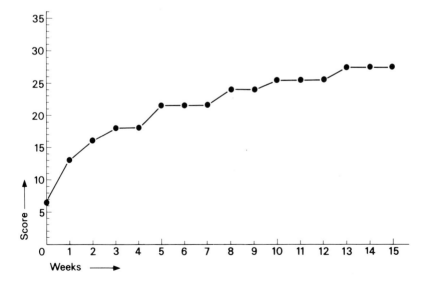

**Fig. 12.4** Recovery curve.

is not so, but it should be possible to develop the concept of merit scores being combined with each new achievement (rather similar to the method of judging used in swimming competitions). Following up a group of such patients over a number of years would eventually identify the significant indicators of good or bad recovery, and a start has been made on this approach with the cohort from Chessington. Once accurate predictions for individuals can be made or accurate recovery times presented, then an intervention in the way of an alternative or added treatment might result in an altered outcome or a change in the graph of the individual.

In the chapter on clinical psychology, reference has already been made to Guttman techniques, in which the hierarchy of recovery is so constructed that it is extremely unlikely to occur out of sequence. This has been applied at Rivermead Rehabilitation Centre to the recovery of motor ability, and Figure 12.5 is not only a chart of the overall function but also an analysis of leg, trunk and arm movements recorded over a three-month period, showing also that this is capable of graphic presentation (Lincoln & Leadbitter 1979). This work was done on stroke patients, but the next use of the techniques was on patients whose brain damage had followed head injury (Whiting & Lincoln 1980) and this has demonstrated that the hierarchy can be attached to the improvement recorded by occupational therapists of the patients in their departments. Thus precise assessment and careful follow-up, together with easy presentation of the information obtained, may be the start of good research methods for the future.

Development of the research referred to is going to be a slow and laborious process, but it seems that only by these exhaustive inquiries can progress be made. Additionally, all this careful analysis is useless if it is not related ultimately to realistic and socially relevant measures of outcome. Tables 12.1 and 12.2 show the outcome measures that have either been used over the last few years or which are now in current use in many centres throughout the world since their inception by the Glasgow workers. For the work of analysis of the Chessington cohort the outcome measures used — accommodation aids supplied, employability, financial situation, personal dependence — were each carefully defined: for example, employability was broken down into five categories and Table 12.4 shows the status of the 103 patients some years after the head injury. From this, correlations can be drawn with other outcome measures; with the initial assessment on entry into the rehabilitation centre; and also with the severity of the initial accident, as judged by duration of unconsciousness, PTA and other factors.

This is not to say that the quality of life of those who are unemployed

| Score 1 or 0                                                               Date: | 18/5 | 21/6 | 20/7 |
|---|---|---|---|
| **GROSS FUNCTION** | | | |
| 1. Sit unsupported | | | |
| 2. Ly. to sitt. on side of bed | | | |
| 3. Sit to st. | | | |
| 4. Transfer from wheelchair to chair twds. unaff. side | | | |
| 5. Transfer from wheelchair to chair twds. aff. side | | | |
| 6. Walk 10 metres independently with an aid | | | |
| 7. Climb stairs independently | | | |
| 8. Walk 10 metres without an aid | | | |
| 9. Walk 5 metres, pick up b.bag from floor, turn & carry back | | | |
| 10. Walk outside 40 metres | | | |
| 11. Walk up and down 4 steps | | | |
| 12. Run 10 metres | | | |
| 13. Hop on affected leg 5 times on the spot | | | |
| TOTAL: | 6 | 11 | 11 |
| **LEG AND TRUNK** | | | |
| 1. Roll to aff. side | | | |
| 2. Roll to unaff. side | | | |
| 3. ½ bridging | | | |
| 4. Sitt. to st. | | | |
| 5. ½ crk.ly; lift aff. leg over side of bed & return it to same posn. | 0 | | |
| 6. St. step unaff. leg on and off block | 0 | | |
| 7. St. tap ground lightly 5 times with unaff. foot | 0 | 0 | 0 |
| 8. Ly. d/flex. ankle with leg flexed | | 0 | 0 |
| 9. Ly. d/flex. ankle with leg ext. | | 0 | 0 |
| 10. St. with aff. hip in neutral position, flex. aff. kn. | | | |
| TOTAL: | 4 | 6 | 6 |
| **ARM** | | | |
| 1. Ly: protract sh. girdle with arm in elevn. | | | |
| 2. Ly: hold ext. arm in elevn. some ext. rot. | | | |
| 3. Flex. & ext. elbow with arms as in 2. | | | |
| 4. Sitt: elb. into side pro. & sup. | | | |
| 5. Reach fwd., pick up large ball with both hands & place down | | | |
| 6. Stretch arm fwd., pick up tennis ball, release on midthigh aff.sideX5 | | | |
| 7. As 6 with pencil X 5. | | | |
| 8. Pick up piece of paper from table in front, release X 5 | | | |
| 9. Cut putty with knife & fork and put into container | | | |
| 10. St: pat large ball on floor with palm of hand X 5 | 0 | 0 | |
| 11. Continuous opp. of thumb & alt. fingers more than 14X in 10 secs. | | | |
| 12. Sup. & pro. onto palm of unaff. hand  20 X in 10 secs. | | | |
| 13. St: hand on wall sh. 90º flex. elb. ext.  Walk round arm. | | | |
| 14. Place string around head, tie bow at back. | | | |
| 15. "Pat-a-cake" 7 X in 15 secs. | | | |
| TOTAL: | 9 | 14 | 15 |

**Fig. 12.5** Rivermead hierarchical assessment.

or unemployable is necessarily unacceptable, either to the patients or
to their relatives, though for some families there is a severe burden.
Quite a few have made new lives for themselves, taken up new skills
and interests, and appear to observers to be leading satisfying lives.
One of the most striking examples was a man who had suffered a head
injury many years prior to assessment and had been out of work and
unemployable for 10 years. He had developed a considerable poetic

Table 12.4    Post-injury employment categories

|  |  |  | Total number of patients |
|---|---|---|---|
| Previous employment | 20 | } Good outcome | 38 |
| Equivalent employment | 18 |  |  |
| Employed, but at poorer status | 15 |  |  |
| Sheltered work | 3 | } Moderate outcome | 23 |
| Training centre | 5 |  |  |
| Unemployed | 19 | } Poor outcome | 37 |
| Unemployable | 18 |  |  |
| N K | 5 |  | 5 |
|  |  |  | 103 |

skill and had published two books of verses which he had sold for the benefit of the Cancer Research Campaign.

On a more practical level, much research is now being undertaken into better methods of coping with problems of incontinence, mobility, spasticity, behavioural problems, so that it is more possible for relatives to care for those who have sustained injury. The role of voluntary bodies and non-governmental organisations also needs mentioning, for this is developing and helping to change for the better the level of handicap within the community. The voluntary sector usually works at local level, and a list of some of the relevant bodies is included in the Appendix. Non-governmental organisations work at international level and aim to coordinate research and development, and to promote the transmission of information both to those who care for the handicapped and to the handicapped themselves. The dissemination of information which is accurate and up to date is done mostly within the United Kingdom through the voluntary societies already referred to, but it is possible that within the next few years this service could be supplemented by the exciting development of Prestel/Viewdata now commercially available with many television sets. This service requires connection to the telephone system, but once this has been established it forms a practical method of getting information for the handicapped into their homes at modest cost. Its controls are simple and capable of being modified even further. Even in its present form, the Prestel/Viewdata system has facilities for leaving messages through the Post Office computer, and as a piece of apparatus the control panel is no more conspicuous than the television set which includes it (Fig. 12.6), and can easily be removed from the television set for remote control operation. Figure 12.7 gives the sort of information than can be stored and reproduced on the set.

Despite all these aids it is likely that some patients will be unable to be cared for at home either because of the severity of their condition or because of the frailty or complete absence of anyone who could

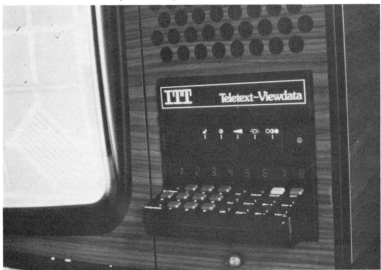

**Fig. 12.6** Prestel/Viewdata set.

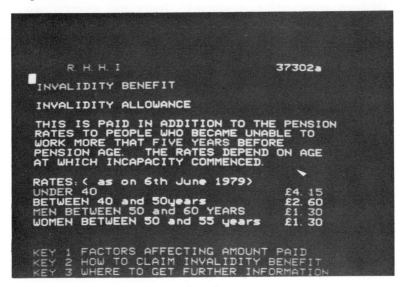

**Fig. 12.7** Sample of Prestel/Viewdata information.

provide care. This happens most commonly when the patients are young and return from hospital or rehabilitation centre to be looked after by ageing parents. The time comes when the situation breaks down and is then replaced by some form of institutional care. At present the provision of such care for the severely brain-damaged is present the provision of such care for the severely brain-damaged is patchy.

There is controversy regarding the role of rehabilitation and its exponents, particularly within the United Kingdom. Many argue that there is no need for such a specialty and that all professions should rehabilitate their own patients. In theory, undoubtedly this is correct. In practice, it does not work, so there does seem to be a need for some centres to undertake research and develop rehabilitation into the future so that at least the techniques which are evolved can be used constructively, and then evaluated objectively.

The role of acute medicine is much easier to recognise but the role of rehabilitation, whatever that may be, is more difficult. Much of the difficulty has been that rehabilitation has stemmed as a discipline from the specialty which was known as physical medicine and whose practitioners used physical treatments to overcome medical problems, often with great success on the part of the patient and practitioner, even if objective evidence as to its effectiveness was, and remains, lacking. Supported with such indifferent evidence, contemporary practitioners of rehabilitation are having to compete with aspects of medicine whose effect is infinitely clearer and in many ways apparently much more cost-effective. It is now possible, though, through the work of the neurophysiologists, to be considerably more optimistic about the future of rehabilitation, particularly for neurological patients.

Sir Henry Osmond Clark in 1946 wrote an article in *The Lancet* about the way in which the services' rehabilitation units had developed. Here are his conclusions:

Many old lessons have been reinforced and strengthened by Royal Air Force experience. (1) Team work is essential; the right man should be hand-picked for the right job; every member of the team has a dual task; the exercise of professional skill and the exercise of a cheerful confident personality. (2) There must be unification of control of the patient from the beginning to the end of the treatment, including regular supervision in rehabilitation centres. The unity is that of control of the team rather than an individual. (3) Good surgery, good rehabilitation are of equal importance. The art as well as the science in good doctoring must be used to inspire and maintain confidence. (4)

Patients are ready to accept treatment in residential rehabilitation centres even after long spells in hospital provided there are adequate facilities for maintaining occasional regular contact with relations. This readiness is not solely due to service disciplines.

These words were written about orthopaedic patients, but when related to head injuries are still apposite. The concept of inpatient rehabilitation centres is opposed partly because of the lack of contemporary experience with them and partly because it is seen as an additional expense to be borne by the authorities for which little benefit can be proven, but Sir Henry's comments about teamwork have a fashionable ring about them and are exemplified at Chessington by the development of an interdisciplinary approach to management of handicap. Figure 10.6 showed a group of patients with severe brain damage undergoing treatment in a gymnasium, which is not unusual, but the therapists included a remedial gymnast, speech therapist, occupational therapist and a nurse. Figure 12.8 shows another part of the same treatment area, though in this situation one-to-one treatment is being offered by both a physiotherapist and a remedial gymnast. Such collaboration has a practical effect for the patient, both in therapeutic terms and also enabling more detailed research to take place. Stichbury et al (1980) have reported on four patients and presented their problems in a way which no single discipline could have undertaken by itself.

It can be argued now that wherever the treatment becomes available for the prolonging of life, a rehabilitation centre should be developed somewhere near since many patients now survive who

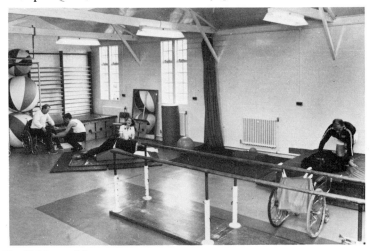

Fig. 12.8 A part of the treatment area.

would have perished and many survive with problems that are severe both physically and mentally. Since the cost of such survival is of the order of £400 000 each, index-linked, effectiveness of rehabilitation really needs to be shown. Some of the new and exciting developments in neurophysiology concerning the recovery of the central nervous system underline the tremendous importance that is going to have to be placed on evaluating and assessing rehabilitation and its effectiveness. However, to be accurate, the benefit that may accrue to the community must be included as part of the equation, otherwise rehabilitation can only be seen to be an expense with no benefit attaching.

REFERENCES

Agerholm M 1978 The classification of personal handicap. Paper given at Medical Commission of Rehabilitation International
Bach-Y-Rita P 1981 Sensory substitution systems. In: Ellis L S, Sedgwick E M, Glanville H J (eds) Rehabilitation of the neurological patient. Blackwell, Oxford
Bach-Y-Rita P 1980 Recovery of function following brain injury: theoretical considerations for brain injury rehabilitation. Huber, Berne
Brodal A 1973 Self-observations and neuro-anatomical considerations after a stroke. Brain 96: 675-694
Jennett B, Bond M 1975 Assessment of outcome after severe brain damage. A practical scale. Lancet i: 480-484
Jennett B 1976 Assessment of the severity of head injury. Journal of Neurology, Neurosurgery and Psychiatry 39: 647-655
Stichbury J, Davenport M, Middleton F 1980 Head-injured patients — a combined therapeutic approach. Physiotherapy, (in press)
Lincoln N B, Leadbitter D 1979 Assessment of motor function in stroke patients. Physiotherapy 65: 48-51
Whiting S E, Lincoln N B 1980 Assessment of activities of daily living in stroke patients. British Journal of Occupational Therapy, Feb 44-46

# Appendix

**List of helpful organisations**
Association of Disabled Professionals
The Stables
73 Pound Road
Banstead
Surrey SM7 2HU

Tel. 07373 52366

A self-help group to improve the rehabilitation of disabled people. Members advise on education/training and employment problems.

British Dyslexia Association
18 The Circus
Bath BA1 2ET

Tel. 0225 20554

Coordinates activities of local associations. Researches into problems of dyslexia and disseminates results of such research.

British Epilepsy Association
Crawthorne House
New Wokingham Road
Wokingham
Berkshire RG11 3AY

Tel. 03446 3122

Northern Ireland Region:
Room 16
16 Claremouth Street Hospital
Belfast BT9 6AQ

Tel. 0232 40491

Provides an information and advisory service.

British Limbless Ex Servicemen's Association
Frankland Moore House
185-197 High Road
Chadwell Heath
Essex RM6 6NA

Tel. 01 590 1124/5

Has local branches. Advises on pensions, employment and welfare matters. Runs two convalescent homes.

British Red Cross
9 Grosvenor Crescent
London SW1X 7EJ

Tel. 01 235 5454

Provides first aid and auxiliary nursing services and many welfare services.

Council and Care for the Elderly
10 Fleet Street
London EC4Y 1BB

Tel. 01 353 1892

Offers financial help and general advice on all matters of concern to people over pension age.

The Disability Alliance
5 Wetherall Gardens
London NW3

Tel. 01 794 1536

Aims to introduce a comprehensive approach to financing disability. Publishes an annual handbook to promote the take-up of existing benefits.

Disabled Drivers Association
Ashwellthrope Hall
Ashwellthrope
Norwich NR16

Tel. 050 841 449

The Association will help and advise physically handicapped people — whether drivers or not — on all mobility matters.

Disabled Drivers' Motor Club Limited
9 Park Parade
Gunnersbury Avenue
London W3 9BD

Tel. 01 993 6454

Offers help and advice on motoring problems.

Disabled Living Foundation
346 Kensington High Street
London W14 8NS

Tel. 01 602 2941

Offers a comprehensive information service; a permanent exhibition of aids and advisory services, with particular reference for problems of incontinence.

Distressed Gentlefolk's Aid Association
Vicarage Gate House
Vicarage Gate
London W8 4AQ

Tel. 01 229 9341

Provides financial help, clothing, comforts and holidays for suitable cases.

Greater London Association for the Disabled (GLAD)
1 Thorpe Close
London W10 5XI

Tel. 01 960 5799

Aims to be an authoritative source on information on local and national welfare legislation. Publishes a directory of clubs in London for physically handicapped people.

Head Injuries Rehabilitation Trust
Birmingham Accident Hospital
Bath Row
Birmingham B15 1NA

All enquiries to the Social Work Department, Tel. 021 643 7041

Facilities include a sheltered workshop, head injuries club and general advice regarding severe head injury problems.

Invalids at Home Trust
23 Farm Avenue
London NW2

Tel. 01 452 2074

Provides money for equipment to enable invalids to stay at home.

John Grooms Association for the Disabled
10 Gloucester Drive
London N4 2LP

Tel. 01 802 7272

Provides care and accommodation. Runs a craft centre with associated homes, and provides holiday accommodation. It also has a housing association promoting provision of purpose-built flats for disabled people.

Motability
Room 550
State House
High Holborn
London WC1R 4SX

Tel. 01 242 9020

A scheme to enable people (whether drivers or passengers) in receipt of a mobility allowance to lease a car by using the allowance.

National Head Injuries Association
17-21 Clumber Avenue
Sherwood Rise
Nottingham NG5 1AG

Tel. 0602 622382

Possum Users' Association
Copper Beech
Parry's Close
Stoke Bishops
Bristol BS9 1AW

Tel. 0272 683596

Assists users of Possum equipment. Also has a qualified full-time welfare officer to visit disabled people and advise on suitable equipment.

Queen Elizabeth's Foundation for the Disabled
Leatherhead
Surrey KT22 0BN

Tel. 037 284 2204

Comprises of four units which provide assessment, further education, vocational training, residential sheltered work, holidays and convalescence.

Royal Association for Disability and Rehabilitation (RADAR)
25 Mortimer Street
London W1N 8AB

Tel. 01 637 5400

Acts as a coordinating body for voluntary groups serving disabled people, and provides information on relevant subjects. Provides publication lists, and publishes Access Guides and other journals.

Scottish Council on Disability
18–19 Claremont Crescent
Edinburgh EH7 4QD

Tel. 031 556 3882

Provides an Information Service, a mobile aids centre and a means of consultation and joint action among voluntary and statutory organisations in Scotland.

Scottish Trust for the Physically Disabled Limited
9 Wheatfield Road
Edinburgh EH11 2PX

Tel. 031 337 5251

Concerned with purpose-built housing with warden supervision and other facilities to enable the physically handicapped to lead as normal a life as possible.

SPOD c/o RADAR
25 Mortimer Street
London W1N 8AB

Tel. 01 637 5400

Aims to promote understanding of the sexual and emotional needs of the disabled. Offers an advisory and counselling service to individuals and arranges training and educational courses on sexual aspects of disability.

**Helpful publications**

Directory for the Disabled
  — a handbook of information and opportunities for
    disabled and handicapped people.
Compiled by A. Darborough and D. Kinrade.

Published in association with RADAR                                £3.60


ABC
  — an ABC of services and information for disabled people.
Written by B. MacMorland.

Published by the Disablement Income Group Charitable Trust, Attlee
  House, Toynbee Hall, 28 Commercial Street, London E1 6LR       £1.00


Access Guides          RADAR
Publication Lists      25 Mortimer Street,
                       London W1N 8AB
                       Tel. 01-637 5400


Green Pages
  — a national/international sourcebook for rehabilitation
    products and services
Available from: Source Book Publications Inc., PO Box 1586, Winter Park,
  Florida 32790, USA
  Tel. 305/628-0545                                              £7.00


The Sexual Side of Handicap
  — a guide for caring professions
By W. Stewart.

Available from Woodhead-Faulkner (Publishers) Limited, 8 Market Passage,
  Cambridge CB2 3PF                                              £8.75
                                                          (p & p inclusive)


Charities Digest

Available from: The Family Welfare Association, 501-503 Kingsland Road,
  Dulston, London E8 4AU
  Tel. 01-254 6251                                               £3.85

INFORMATION CENTRES FOR DISABLED PEOPLE

**North**

*Regional Representative*
Newcastle upon Tyne Disabled Information and Advisory Service
MEA House
Ellison Place
Newcastle

Tel. 0632 23617

Hull Disability Rights Advisory Service
Room 4
The Central Methodist Mission
King Edward Street
Hull

Tel. 0482 22634

DIAL Leeds
Halton Moor Information Centre
Neville Road
Leeds 15

Tel. 0532 608901

Disablement Information Bureau, Durham
26 St Margaret's Court
Durham DM1 4QY

Tel. 0385 62127

**North Midlands**

*Regional Representative*
DIAL Derbyshire
Cressy Fields
Cressy Road
Alfreton
Derbyshire

Tel. 077 383 3220

DIAL Rotherham
23 Holdesness Drive
Swallownest
Sheffield

Tel. 0742 874106

DIAL Sheffield
751 Ecckshall Road
Sheffield

Tel. 0742 861186

DIAL Nottingham
14 Notintone Place
Sneinton Dale
Nottingham

Tel. 0602 55656

## North West

*Regional Representative*
DIAL Bangor
31 Strand Street
Bangor
Gwynedd

Tel. 0248 52197

Manchester Telephone Advisory Bureau
c/o Community Development Section
Solway House
Aytonn Street
Manchester

Tel. 061 228 2111

Wirral Association for the Disabled Information Service
52 Bertram Drive
Meols
Wirral
Merseyside

Tel. 051 632 2857

## Midlands

*Regional Representative*
DIAL Coventry
26 Lechlade Close
Henley Green
Coventry
Warwickshire

Tel. Henley Green 0203 611101

DIAL Daventry
18 Townsend Road
Woodford Halse
Daventry
Northants

Tel. 0327 61122

DIAL Leicester
6 St Martins
Leicester

Tel. 0533 303431

DIAL Corby
The Stonehouse
South Road
Corby
Northants

Tel. 053 66 4642

Birmingham Handicapped Children's Service
Room 104
102 Edmund Street
Birmingham 3

Tel. 021 235 2475

DIAL Wolverhampton
Neighbourhood Advice Centre
43 Church Street
Bilston
West Midlands

## London and East

*Regional Representative*
Wandsworth Disabled Advice Service
Atheldene Centre
305 Garrett Lane
London SW18

Tel. 01 870 7437

Barnet Disability Information Service
Flightwave Day Centre
1 The Concourse
Graham Park Estate
Colindale
London NW9

Tel. 01 205 5803/4

Newham Handicap Help Line
c/o 88 High Street South
London E6

Tel. 01 471 7188

Ask Norwich
Gaffers Cottage
Grange Farm
Spixworthy
Norfolk

Tel. 0603 51061

DIAL Medway
c/o 89 Rock Avenue
Gillingham
Kent

Tel. 0634 576661

## South West

*Regional Representative*
Exeter Disability Rights Advisory Service
3 Palace Gate
Exeter
Devon

Tel. 0392 59336

Truro Hi Line
c/o Cornwall Association for the Disabled
56 Lemon Street
Truro
Cornwall

Tel. 0872 2314

Cardiff Disabled Information Service
45 Port Place
Cardiff

Tel. 0222 398058

Bristol Disabled Advice Centre
Westmorland House
104 Stokes Croft
Bristol

Tel. 0272 423908

## WHERE TO SEE AIDS

The following centres have displays where a selection of aids for the handicapped may be seen and tried out. Visitors should contact the aids centres before visiting as an appointment is usually necessary. Some centres also run an enquiries service for telephone or written queries.

### Aid centres

*Birmingham*
>Disabled Living Centre
84 Suffolk Street
Birmingham B1

Tel. 021 643 0980

*Caerphilly*
>Aids and Information Centre
Wales Council for the Disabled
Llys Ifor
Crescent Road
Caerphilly
Mid Glamorgan CF8 1XL

Tel. 0222 869224

*Leicester*
>Medical Aids Department
British Red Cross Society
76 Clarendon Park Road
Leicester LE2 3AD

Tel. 0533 700747

*Liverpool*

Merseyside Aids Centre
Yonens Way
East Prescott Road
Liverpool 14

Tel. 051228 9221

*London*

Disabled Living Foundation
Aids and Information Centre
346 Kensington High Street
London W14 8NS

Tel. 01 602 2491

*Manchester*

Cripples Help Society
26 Blackfriars Street
Manchester M3 5BE

Tel. 061 832 3678

*Newcastle upon Tyne*

Newcastle upon Tyne Council for the Disabled
Aids Centre and Information Service
Mea House, Ellison Place
Newcastle upon Tyne NE1 8XS

Tel. 0682 23617

*Southampton*

Hampshire Area Health Authority
Southampton General Hospital
Shirley
Southampton SO9 4XY

Tel. 0703 777222 ext. 3122 or 2414

*Stockport*

Aids/Assessment Unit
Stockport Area Health Authority
Stepping Hill Hospital
Stockport

Tel. 061 483 1010 ext. 207

*Wakefield*
   National Demonstration Centre
   Pinderfields Hospital
   Pinderfields
   Wakefield
   Yorkshire

   Tel. 0924 75217 ext. 2510 or 2263


**Mobile aid centres**
These are travelling exhibitions of aids which visit various parts of the
country. Contact the organisations for details of dates and places to be visited.
   Mobile Aids Centre
   Scottish Information Service for the Disabled
   18/19 Claremont Crescent
   Edinburgh EH7 4QD

   Tel. 031 556 3882

   Travelling Exhibition of Aids
   Royal Association for Disability and Rehabilitation (RADAR)
   25 Mortimer Street
   London W1 8AB

   Tel. 01 637 5400

   Visiting Aids Centre
   Spastic Society
   12 Park Crescent
   London W1

   Tel. 01 636 5020

# Index